# A PEDIATRIC RESIDENT POCKET GUIDE

# MAKING THE MOST OF MORNING REPORT

# PEDIATRICS, CHILD AND ADOLESCENT HEALTH

## JOAV MERRICK – SERIES EDITOR –

NATIONAL INSTITUTE OF CHILD HEALTH AND HUMAN DEVELOPMENT,
MINISTRY OF SOCIAL AFFAIRS, JERUSALEM, ISRAEL

**Child and Adolescent Health Yearbook 2012**
*Joav Merrick (Editor)*
2012. ISBN: 978-1-61942-788-4

**Child Health and Human Development Yearbook 2011**
*Joav Merrick (Editor)*
2012. ISBN: 978-1-61942-969-7

**Tropical Pediatrics: A Public Health Concern of International Proportions**
*Richard R Roach,
Donald E Greydanus, Dilip R Patel,
Douglas N Homnick
and Joav Merrick (Editors)*
2012. ISBN: 8-1-61942-831-7

**Developmental Issues in Chinese Adolescents**
*Daniel TL Shek, Rachel CF Sun and
Joav Merrick (Editors)*
2012. ISBN: 978-1-62081-262-4

**Positive Youth Development: Theory, Research and Application**
*Daniel TL Shek, Rachel CF Sun
and Joav Merrick (Editors)*
2012. ISBN: 978-1-62081-305-8

**Understanding Autism Spectrum Disorder: Current Research Aspects**
*Ditza A Zachor and
Joav Merrick (Editors)*
2012. ISBN: 978-1-62081-353-9

**Positive Youth Development: A New School Curriculum to Tackle Adolescent Developmental Issues**
*Hing Keung Ma, Daniel TL Shek and
Joav Merrick (Editors)*
2012. ISBN: 978-1-62081-384-3

**Transition from Pediatric to Adult Medical Care**
*David Wood, John G Reiss, Maria E
Ferris, Linda R Edwards and Joav
Merrick (Editors)*
2012. ISBN: 978-1-62081-409-3

**Guidelines for the Healthy Integration of the Ill Child in the Educational System: Experience from Israel**
*Yosefa Isenberg*
2013. ISBN: 978-1-62808-350-7

**Chinese Adolescent Development: Economic Disadvantages, Parents and Intrapersonal Development**
*Daniel TL Shek, Rachel CF Sun and Joav Merrick (Editors)*
2013. ISBN: 978-1-62618-622-4

**University and College Students: Health and Development Issues for the Leaders of Tomorrow**
*Daniel TL Shek, Rachel CF Sun and Joav Merrick (Editors)*
2013. ISBN: 978-1-62618-586-9

**Adolescence and Behavior Issues in a Chinese Context**
*Daniel TL Shek, Rachel CF Sun and Joav Merrick (Editors)*
2013. ISBN: 978-1-62618-614-9

**Advances in Preterm Infant Research**
*Jing Sun, Nicholas Buys and Joav Merrick*
2013. ISBN: 978-1-62618-696-5

**Internet Addiction: A Public Health Concern in Adolescence**
*Artemis Tsitsika, Mari Janikian, Donald E. Greydanus, Hatim A. Omar and Joav Merrick (Editors)*
2013. ISBN: 978-1-62618-925-6

**Promotion of Holistic Development of Young People in Hong Kong**
*Daniel TL Shek, Tak Yan Lee and Joav Merrick (Editors)*
2013. ISBN: 978-1-62808-019-3

**Human Developmental Research: Experience from Research in Hong Kong**
*Daniel TL Shek, Cecilia Ma, Yu Lu and Joav Merrick (Editors)*
2013. ISBN: 978-1-62808-166-4

**Chronic Disease and Disability in Childhood**
*Joav Merrick*
2013. ISBN: 978-1-62808-865-6

**Break the Cycle of Environmental Health Disparities: Maternal and Child Health Aspects**
*Leslie Rubin and Joav Merrick (Editors)*
2013. ISBN: 978-1-62948-107-4

**Environmental Health Disparities in Children: Asthma, Obesity and Food**
*Leslie Rubin and Joav Merrick (Editors)*
2013. ISBN: 978-1-62948-122-7

**Environmental Health: Home, School and Community**
*Leslie Rubin and Joav Merrick (Editors)*
2013. ISBN: 978-1-62948-155-5

# A PEDIATRIC RESIDENT POCKET GUIDE

# MAKING THE MOST OF MORNING REPORT

## ARTHUR N. FEINBERG

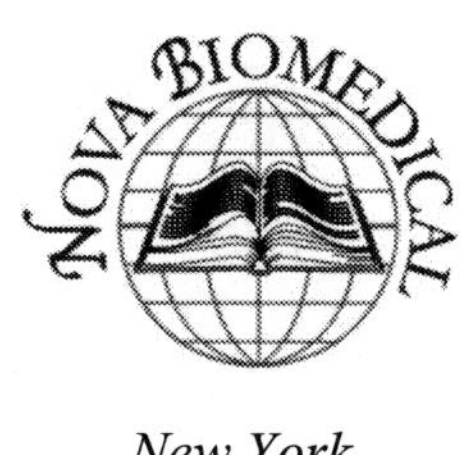

New York

**NOTICE TO THE READER**

The Publisher has taken reasonable care in the preparation of this book, but makes no expressed or implied warranty of any kind and assumes no responsibility for any errors or omissions. No liability is assumed for incidental or consequential damages in connection with or arising out of information contained in this book. The Publisher shall not be liable for any special, consequential, or exemplary damages resulting, in whole or in part, from the readers' use of, or reliance upon, this material. Any parts of this book based on government reports are so indicated and copyright is claimed for those parts to the extent applicable to compilations of such works.

Independent verification should be sought for any data, advice or recommendations contained in this book. In addition, no responsibility is assumed by the publisher for any injury and/or damage to persons or property arising from any methods, products, instructions, ideas or otherwise contained in this publication.

This publication is designed to provide accurate and authoritative information with regard to the subject matter covered herein. It is sold with the clear understanding that the Publisher is not engaged in rendering legal or any other professional services. If legal or any other expert assistance is required, the services of a competent person should be sought. FROM A DECLARATION OF PARTICIPANTS JOINTLY ADOPTED BY A COMMITTEE OF THE AMERICAN BAR ASSOCIATION AND A COMMITTEE OF PUBLISHERS.

Additional color graphics may be available in the e-book version of this book.

**Library of Congress Cataloging-in-Publication Data**

ISBN: 978-1-63482-141-4
Library of Congress Control Number: 2015931767

*Published by Nova Science Publishers, Inc.† New York*

# CONTENTS

# DEDICATION AND ACKNOWLEDGMENTS

I dedicate this book to every single resident in whose training I have played a part. After twenty years in private practice, I felt the need to shift gears and work more closely with residents. I went into this with the idea in mind that I was going to teach them, but little did I know how much they were going to teach me. The mutual "back-and-forth" has truly sustained me.

Over the years I have particularly grown to love morning report with all the factual, practical and humanitarian discussions that evolve from them. I have witnessed the evolution of its format over the years and strongly feel it is one of our most important venues for resident education. Hence, much of this treatise has been based on my morning report experience.

As I have broached the topic of retirement over the years, many residents have said "could you at least wait until I graduate?" I take this as a supreme compliment, but find that if I continue on like this, I will never be able to retire. Pulling on the other end is the aging process, and the need to do many things before it is too late such as seeing more of the world and spending time with my wife Marilyn, children, Lisa and Daniel, and of course my grandchildren, Ruthie, Peanut, Jellybean and Bubba. Practicing medicine is always a calling, and a daunting one at that. Thus, I feel that retiring from medicine should come before my residents and younger colleagues tell me, politely or otherwise, that it is time to go.

I sincerely hope that all my years of practice have left some impact on those I have helped train. If so, this manual will serve as my small legacy to them and subsequent learners. I fully expect that future generations of residents will add to, revise and greatly improve this work.

This book is not really a simple "how to" manual, nor is it laden with medical facts, but rather a digestible distillation of 45 years of clinical experience. As emphasized throughout, it serves as a skeletal framework for the resident on which to add knowledge and experience and as a springboard for discussion of medial decision-making. Two standard works were helpful in developing this project: Bates' Pocket Guide to Physical Examination and History Taking, Wolters, Kluwer, Heath/Lippincott Williams and Wilkins, 2013 and The Pediatric Diagnostic Examination, Greydanus, Feinberg, Patel and Homnick Editors, Mc Graw-Hill New York 2008. Many of the philosophical points were gleaned, not only from experience (my mentors and some hard knocks), but well-crystallized in the most important book, "How Doctors Think" by Dr. Jerome Groopman, Houghton Mifflin Co. 2007. This book is a "must read" for all physicians at all levels of experience.

I give special thanks to senior residents Zahra Benn who planted the idea for this project and to Megan Sikkema for her most scrupulous editing.

# INTRODUCTION

Our main goal is to introduce the beginning student or pediatric resident to a systematic method of medical decision making. We divide the manual into three basic sections:

1)  History-taking
2)  Physical examination
3)  Medical reasoning

It is important to note that the purpose of this book is NOT to teach everything there is to know about every possible medical diagnosis, but rather to establish a framework for reasoning out a problem. We assume that as the learners read about and experience many more encounters over their training period they will be able to apply the facts to this basic framework. Thus, it is important to note that the history-taking and physical examination, first and second sections specifically do NOT mention any diagnoses. Their main purpose is to present the full array of data that needs to be gathered. Note the insertion of several clinical tricks of the trade to help gain accurate data. The third section, medical reasoning will take the reader through the thought process of arriving at a diagnosis. It addresses sifting and winnowing through large amounts of data: interpretation of history, what questions to ask, what questions may or may not be pertinent to the situation at hand, making initial hypotheses and testing them with information from a physical examination. We discuss what to examine based on the history, interpreting the remaining data, re-evaluating hypotheses, re-thinking them and narrowing them further, ideally (but not always) into a unifying hypothesis. If necessary, we discuss the use of laboratory and imaging as further means to test hypotheses. We then discuss making treatment plans with the idea forefront in the mind that the hypothesis still may indeed be wrong and have to be revised.

The narrowing-down process is critical and necessary for the rational practice of medicine and the techniques are often referred to as "heuristics" (short-cuts). They are most helpful, but are certainly not infallible. We therefore discuss pitfalls in clinical diagnosis in order to keep the reader keenly aware of the fact that hypotheses are in need of constant review and revision if necessary.

We present two illustrative and simple cases as journeys through the medical reasoning process. As the learner progresses, he/she will learn to navigate through more difficult cases, However, our more simple cases provide the tools to use for the more complex ones.

It is our hope that early on in medical training the learners will appreciate the importance of good histories and physical examinations and how to interpret them. They will find that much of the information gathered in this manner will serve them well and lead to more judicious and appropriate usage of technology to arrive at diagnoses.

# Chapter 1

# Gathering data: Taking a pediatric history

## Basic Outline

I.  Pre-interview preparation
    A.  **Review chart**
    B.  Have knowledge of patient and/or caregiver's background (developmental/cognitive level, literacy, sophistication, beliefs, concerns, fears etc.)
II. Introduction and establishing rapport
    A.  Introduce self
    B.  Put patient/caregiver at ease. If you have knowledge of interviewee's interests, hobbies, etc.; touching on this briefly may help.
    C.  Take a seat opposite patient; maintain equal level of eye-contact. It patient is an infant or child, it may be best to start with patient in parent's lap and, if necessary, maintain this for the entire encounter. Be aware of distractibility of small children and play it to the hilt!
    D.  Explain the purpose of the visit (work with patient, to establish an agenda)
    E.  Maintain confidentiality
III. The historian-centered interviews – as a rule, always start with open-ended questions and let the patient do the talking. Do not interrupt. Follow with questions for clarification, quantification and addition. In

extreme instances of loquaciousness or disorganization on the part of
the patient, some re-direction may be appropriate.

   A.   Chief Complaint
        1.   Always in the patient's own words
        2.   The OPQRST mnemonic:
             O – Onset
             P – Provocative or palliative measures
             Q – Quality of the problem
             R – Region involved, including radiation
             S – Severity of the problem
             T – Temporal pattern of the problem
        3.   Clarification
        a.   Quality - May have to offer choices regarding OPQRST
             for the patient to select, if not clear. For example, further
             description of pain: sharp, dull, deep. Also, offer other
             pertinent provocative or palliative measures, if not
             mentioned. May need clarification of a word, e g: does
             "dizzy" mean you are, or the room is spinning? Patient
             logs of a problem are often helpful to clarify timing of a
             symptom.
        b.   Quantity – Examples: How much blood? How much
             urine? How frequently? Pain scale
        c.   Associated problems – ask first in open-ended manner.
             Closed questions may be considered "leading." However,
             specific questions answered properly can serve as useful
             "pertinent negatives." For example, the clinician may
             want to know if the patient's vomiting is associated with
             diarrhea, constipation, jaundice, etc.
   B.   Past history
        1.  Medical
        2.  Surgical
        3.  Allergies, intolerances
        4.  Medications
        5.  Preventive: immunizations, home safety precautions,
            screening
        6.  Birth history, neonatal history
   C.   Family history

    1.   Obtain ages and health status of parents, siblings and children, including illnesses and causes of death if present.

    2.   Systems-related illnesses in family members such as diabetes, hypertension, arthritis, cancer, cardiac, pulmonary, renal, endocrine, neurologic, psychiatric disorder

    3.   Hone in on more specific disorders, e g, thyroid disease, asthma.

D.  Personal and social history

    1.   Demographic data (age, gender, race, ethnic)

    2.   Socioeconomic status

    3.   Support systems

    4.   Educational level

    5.   Important life experiences, hobbies, religious beliefs

    6.   Lifestyle – smoking, alcohol and drug consumption, diet and exercise, safety and health precautions, use of alternative and complementary medicine, travels, exposures (illnesses, toxins)

E.  Review of systems

    1.   Head-to-toe

    2.   Yes-no

    3.   System-by-system

F.  Developmental history

    1. Gross motor

    2. Fine motor

    3. Adaptive

    4. Language

    5. Personal-social

# TRICKS OF THE TRADE

## Basic interviewing skills

Interview is patient-centered. However, there has to be shared partnering based on mutual respect.

    Obligations of provider:

Be prepared – review the chart!

Put patient/caregiver at ease (physical comfort, privacy, maintain eye-level)

Set goals for the interview (patient-centered)

Ask open-ended questions initially

Listen actively to the responses – try not to interrupt

Be empathetic by tending to all clues patient may provide, both verbal and non-verbal


Empower patient/caregiver by:


Acknowledging and understanding the patient's perspectives (have understanding of patient's background and belief-systems)

Following patient's leads

Sharing information with patient in a way he/she can understand (minimize medical jargon, even if the patient is a physician)

Validating patient's thoughts and feelings

Identify problematic patient cues and try to understand from where they arose

Recognizing lack of patient understanding by repeating questions, prolonged silences, even tacit smiling

Understanding cues of disbelief/dissatisfaction such as head-shaking, sighing, refusal to conclude interview, reluctance to accept recommendations ("yeah-but…" really means "no.")

Have a discrete "question and answer" period encouraging and accepting all questions from the patient and allowing adequate time for them

Feeling certain patient understands the information. Interpret and recapitulate frequently; ask patient to answer pertinent questions.

Feeling certain patient is not telling you what you want to hear. Some cultures do dictate subservience in this situation.

Do not have your mind made up until the conclusion of the visit

Self-reflection

Understanding own values

Understanding patient's background and origin of their values

Do not foist your values on the patient. If your values and the patient's do clash, or if you think the patient is doing something you perceive as "wrong" it is best not to say they are "wrong", but rather to explore alternative means of dealing with the situation ("It seems like you are frustrated and what you are trying; hitting your child, is not working. Why don't we try something else?")

One exception: if a patient is doing something that is illegal or dangerous to self or others, then this should be pointed out.

After the interview, explore with yourself how it went and what you might have done differently.

## Obligations of patient

Be prepared – have history thought out previously

Stick to the agenda. Do not go off on too many tangents. Answer questions relevant to what is asked. Have your questions prepared and be ready to ask them during the "question and answer" period.

Try to be as informed as much as possible about your situation, share with physician your "on-line" sources, but be sure to be receptive to your provider's interpretation of the information.

Do not come with your mind made up. The interview is a collaborative process to mutually work out a solution.

All interviews are two-way. Feel free to ask physician for clarification at any time. Never feel intimidated if you do not understand a question.

There is no such thing as a "stupid" question. Feel free to ask and, if not clear or satisfied with the answer, please express concerns, albeit politely. Be certain you have had all your questions answered to your satisfaction.

## The challenging interview

The silent patient – Is the patient shy? Is the patient offended? Is the patient angry, or depressed?

The confusing patient – Is the story making sense? Does any of the content seem recognizable enough to give you a lead as to where to investigate next? If it does, is it presented in such a disorganized manner as to be confusing? Could the patient be impaired due to mental illness, intoxication or intellectual disability?

The chatty/repetitive patient – May have to ask questions to redirect the conversation to what is relevant. Could the repetition be due to dementia?

The crying patient – Do express your understanding. ("I know how difficult this is for you.") You may have to redirect the conversation after calming patient down.

The angry or hostile patient – Validate their feelings and express understanding as to why they could be angry ("you had a long wait", "no one has been able to figure out your problem.") It is OK to say "I'm sorry" for something that happened in the past. Always ask how we can fix this problem. Keep your composure and never get angry back at the patient. If the patient will not calm down or makes threats, it is then appropriate to notify security.

The patient with a language barrier – Many practices have direct contact to an interpreter service. Have a list of employees in your organization who speak other languages. Caveat re using family members as interpreters: Sometimes a relative may know of the patient's vulnerabilities and will avoid translating some of your questions exactly.

The patient with hearing impairment – Keep room well-lit, sit with eyes at same level as the patient's and faces the patient to facilitate lip-reading. Be sure to remove all ambient noise. Do not yell at the patient. Use American Sign Language (ASL) if this is the means of communication. There is a video service for the hearing impaired where a translator can receive ASL from the patient and speak to the provider.

The visually impaired patient – Keep room well lit and first orient patient to the room's geography.

The patient with multiple issues – If this is the primary reason for the visit let them talk it out as this will often help. If other issues are raised at the close of the visit (Oh, by the way, Doc") this could cause potential backups in the daily flow and it may be necessary to schedule another visit to address these questions.


## SENSITIVE CONVERSATIONS


### Domestic violence

It is always important to ask all patients if they feel safe at home. It can be helpful to know this when asking further questions. Many times a teenager will say "My father/mother would kill me if he/she ever finds this out." Sometimes it can be difficult to determine if this is real or imagined, but if you can sense initially that the patient feels safe at home and the parents seem reasonable to you, there may be less risk for harm. If you feel there is low risk for harm in the home, explore with the patient what his/her fears are. Nonetheless, avoid betraying confidences unless you are convinced that the patient is at risk for doing harm to self or others.

## Sexual history

In teenagers, this subject can be even more difficult because it may potentially involve both patient and parent(s). It is always preferable to interview the patient without the parents and emphasize the importance of confidentiality. In most cases, this happens easily. If a parent or parents are adamant about being in the room explain that confidentiality is the best way to get truthful answers. It is important to ask questions neither too generally ("How's your sex life." "Fine"), or too specifically "(When was the last time you had oral sex"), as the patient may feel like he/she is being interrogated. It is important not to belie your sexual opinions and values, and do keep in mind that teenagers are often hypersensitive to body language. In spite of beliefs that may have been instilled in us, sexual orientation is not a consciously adopted perverse lifestyle, and all providers must understand this. Ask questions in a neutral manner. "Have you been sexually attracted to anyone?" If yes, then ask "Same or different sex?" It is always appropriate to point out to a patient that promiscuity and other sexual practices have serious risks; however, moralizing will accomplish nothing and will likely work negatively.

Always inquire into sexual abuse. You might preface this by stating that this is routine and not personally directed to the patient. Start general and work toward specific, if warranted. "Have you ever had any negative sexual experiences?" "Has anyone ever touched you in a way that made you feel uncomfortable?"

Note red flags for abuse, both physical and sexual

- Unexplained or poorly explained injuries
- Delay in getting treatment
- Domineering partner during an office interview
- Repeated STIs or pregnancies at a young age
- Disproportionate fear of genital examination

## Drug abuse, smoking and alcohol

Teenagers may not be forthright about these subjects. Sometimes it is more denial than outright lying. Most people will underreport their tobacco and alcohol consumption. It is often helpful to broach the topic through the "back door." "Do you have any friends who smoke or drink?" If the answer is "yes" then ask if they have ever offered it to you or pressured you to use it. Ask in a non-threatening way if they have been tempted to or actually smoked or drank alcohol. The conversation may lead to more honest answers. Always look at the patient's body language to sense if they are feeling defensive (bracing one's self, looking scared, losing eye contact) and re-emphasize confidentiality as often as necessary. If the patient admits to using alcohol, then use the CAGE questions (Cutting down, Annoyance when asked, Guilt feelings and Eye-opener).


## Mental health

This can be quite dicey, because each patient brings to the table multiple cultural, familial and personal opinions on this subject.

Questioning for depression and suicide is critical in children and adolescents. Suicidal ideation, intent and all attempts must be taken seriously. It is important to assess if the patient is feeling that way, now, because emergent action may be necessary. Moreover, especially in an older child or young teenager, do not automatically dismiss an argument with a parent over doing homework and a subsequent suicide attempt as "mere drama." Even if that were the case, younger individuals often lack the judgment to realize that there still can be unintended consequences of their action.

Always ask questions from general to specific. "Do you feel OK, emotionally?" "How do you feel about yourself?" "Have you ever sought help with this?" "Would you like to get some help?" Once the patient seems to be opening up, it is appropriate for them to fill out a depression screening test (PSQ).

# Gathering data: The pediatric anatomic physical examination observation, palpation, percussion, auscultation

## Basic Outline

I. Gestalt (all 5 senses) – quick
- A. Observation (visual, auditory, olfactory, gustatory and tactile)
    1. Mental status, alertness, demeanor, communication (visual, auditory)
    2. Morphology (visual, tactile)
    3. Nourishment (visual, tactile)
    4. Hydration (visual, tactile)
    5. Olfactory (sweet, musky, fetid, ammonia)
    6. Sounds (respiratory, evaluation of cry)
    7. Gustatory (patient could taste salty, but do not start out eating kids, as it makes a bad first impression)

II. Vital signs
- A. Observation
    1. Respirations
    2. Measurement of height and weight and head circumference with percentiles and growth chart plots
    3. Pulse oximetry
    4. Temperature

    B.  Palpation
- 1.  Pulse rate, quality

    C.  Auscultation
- 1.  Pulse rate, quality
- 2.  Blood pressure oscillometry vs. sphygmomanometry

III.  Head and neck

    A.  Observation
- 1.  Size
- 2.  Morphology
  - a.  Shape
  - b.  Symmetry
  - c.  Prominences
  - d.  Masses
- 3.  Transillumination, skull, sinuses

    B.  Palpation
- 1.  Fontanelle
- 2.  Sutures
- 3.  Masses

    C.  Percussion
- 1.  Tympanitic?
- 2.  Dullness

    D.  Auscultation
- 1.  Bruits
- 2.  Breath sounds

IV.  Eyes

    A.  Observation
- 1.  Overall morphology
  - a.  Size
  - b.  Shape
  - c.  Color
- 2.  Lacrimation
- 3.  Pupillary shape and responses
  - a.  "PERRLA"
- 4.  Movements
  - a.  Spontaneous
  - b.  Extraocular muscle function
- 5.  Sclerae
  - a.  Color (red, yellow, blue, pigmentation)
- 6.  Cornea

        a.   Size
        b.   Clarity
        c.   Ophthalmoscopy with and without blue light
      7.  Fundi
        a.   Ophthalmoscopy
    B.  Palpation
      1.  Size
      2.  Intraocular tension

V.  Ears, nose and throat
    Ears
    A.  Observation
      1. Visual
      2. Olfactory
  Nose
    A.  Observation
      1. Visual
      2. Olfactory
    B.  Palpation
  Throat
    A.  Observation
       1. Visual
       2. Olfactory

VI.  Thorax (external, pulmonary and cardiac)
    A.  Observation
    B.  Palpation
    C.  Percussion
    D.  Auscultation

VII. Abdomen anal and rectal
    A.  Observation
    B.  Palpation
    C.  Percussion
    D.  Auscultation

VIII. Genitalia (male, female, the pelvic examination)
    A.  Observation
    B.  Palpation

IX.  Extremities (non-musculoskeletal)
    A.  Observation
    B.  Palpation

X.  Musculoskeletal – general

      A.  Observation
      B.  Palpation
  XI.  Musculoskeletal – sports medicine
      A.  Observation
      B.  Palpation
  XII.  Neurologic (Consider full examination including observation, palpation, percussion and auscultation to help determine if there are neurologic manifestations of a systemic condition)
  XIII.  Dermatologic (Consider full examination including observation, palpation, percussion and auscultation to help determine if there is a dermatologic manifestation of a systemic condition)

## EXPANSION OF THE BASIC OUTLINE

Gestalt (all 5 senses) – quick overview of WDWN WH NAD (Well-developed, well-nourished, well hydrated, no apparent distress)

**Observation** (visual, auditory, olfactory, gustatory and tactile)

Are there obvious dysmorphic findings or malformations? Is there symmetry or asymmetry to them? What do the findings feel like (hard, soft, fluctuant, mobile, uniform)? Group them together by anatomic region. Are there obvious external lesions of the skin? Are they traumatic? Is there evidence of body fluids on or near the patient?

Are there any sounds coming from the patient, specifically associated with respiration? What is the quality of the voice or cry?

Are there any noticeable odors from the patient? Are they sweet, sour, musky, fetid or ammoniac?

Nourishment (visual, tactile)

Body habitus: Is the weight commensurate with the height or length? What is the amount and distribution of fat on the patient? Does the skin appear tight or flaccid?

Hydration (visual, tactile)

How moist are the mucus membranes? Are there tears? How alert is the patient? Is the skin tight or flaccid?

Mental_status (alertness, demeanor, visual and auditory communication)

Is the patient comfortable? Are there any visual signs of discomfort, distress or pain? Is the patient awake and alert, sleepy, obtunded, comatose, irritable? Do these signs change when the patient is stimulated? Is the patient consolable if irritable? Does the patient come to attention if sleepy or obtunded; to what extent? How is the interchange of conversation? Are the patient's responses appropriate?

How well does the patient make contact with you? Is there eye contact? How good is verbal communication? Is the verbal level of communication in keeping with development (single words, short sentences, full sentences, concepts and ideas, subtlety and nuances)?

Body language is very important. Is the patient "in sync" with you (open posture, interacting) or trying to avoid you (averted gaze, closed posture, texting, playing video games)? Is he/she angry or annoyed? Is the patient happy or sad? Is the patient phlegmatic, hyperactive or manic?

Vital Signs Temperature, Pulse, Respiration, Blood Pressure, pulse oximetry, height, weight, head circumference, body mass index (BMI) and pain assessment

## OBSERVATION

Pulse: Are heartbeats visible on the chest wall?

Respirations: rate, depth, degree of distress, if any, determined by retractions, use of accessory muscles of respiration, nasal flaring.

Pulse oximetry: Is the patient pale or cyanotic? Make hypothesis and test it by using a pulse oximeter.

Height, weight, head circumference and BMI: Make initial visual assessments and back up with measurement. If the measurement is not congruent with your initial assessment, re-measure!

## PALPATION

Temperature: does the patient feel warm or cold? Is the skin dry or sweaty? Make hypothesis and test it by using a valid measurement of core-temperature detection, usually a digital thermometer, orally or rectally, or an accurate

 *Arthur N Feinberg*

axillary temperature for at least 3 minutes with axilla totally closed, admitting no environmental air.

Pulse: rate (fast or slow with regard to age norms), rhythm (regular, irregular); if irregular is it random or does it have a pattern, e. g. duplet, or triplet? Does it vary with respirations? Is the pulse weak or strong?

# AUSCULTATION

Pulse: use auscultation to confirm your impressions on palpation

Blood Pressure:

Korotkoff sounds

Be certain cuff is of appropriate size for the patient. The bladder of the cuff should be at least 20% wider than the diameter of the limb and at least half as long as the circumference of the limb.

I. A loud clear cut snapping tone $\qquad$ $P_{cuff} = P_{systolic}$

II. A succession of murmurs $\qquad$ $P_{diastolic} \ll P_{cuff} < P_{systolic}$

III. The disappearance of the murmurs and the appearance of a tone resembling to a degree the first phase, but less well-marked

$P_{diastolic} < P_{cuff} \ll P_{systolic}$

IV. Muffling of taps $\qquad$ $P_{diastolic} \leq P_{cuff}$

V. Silence $\qquad$ $P_{diastolic} \geq P_{cuff}$

# RECOMMENDATIONS FOR BLOOD PRESSURE MEASUREMENT

| RECOMMENDATION | COMMENT |
|---|---|
| Patient should be seated comfortably with back supported, legs uncrossed and upper arm bared | Diastolic pressure is higher in the seated position whereas systolic pressure is higher in the supine position<br><br>An unsupported back may increase diastolic pressure, crossing the legs may increase systolic pressure |

| RECOMMENDATION | COMMENT |
|---|---|
| Patient's arm should be supported at heart level | If the upper arm is below the level of the right atrium, the readings will be too high. If the upper arm is above the heart level, the readings will be too low<br><br>If the arm is unsupported and held up by the patient, pressure will be higher |
| Cuff bladder should encircle 80% or more of the patient's arm circumference and cover at least 2/3 of the upper arm | An undersized cuff increases errors in measurement |
| Mercury column should be deflated at 2 to 3 mm /sec | Deflations rates > 2mm/sec can cause systolic pressure to appear lower and the diastolic pressure to appear higher |
| The 1$^{st}$ and last audible sounds should be recorded as the systolic and diastolic pressure respectively. Measurements should be given to the nearest 2 mm Hg | |
| Neither the patient nor the person taking the measurement should talk during the procedure | Talking during the procedure may cause deviations in the measurement |

Interpretation of blood pressure: Consult tables for BP percentiles

# HEAD AND NECK EXAMINATION

## Observation

Head

Size: Plot on growth curve. Determine percentile for age. Follow trend of head growth over time

Morphology:

Is the head shaped normally?

Is there symmetry or asymmetry?

Is there a pattern to the symmetry or asymmetry? Does the asymmetry appear to be anatomic or positional?

Are there any masses or prominences? Are they midline or lateral?
Are there any defects or lesions on the skin?
Transillumination: Does the skull "light up?"

Neck
Size and morphology:
Is it long or short or proportionate?
Is the circumference proportionate?
Evaluate for symmetry and posture
Evaluate for masses, size, shape, induration, location
Are there defects or lesions on the skin?

Technique for thyroid examination

1)   Observe at rest
2)   Observe as patient swallows water
3)   Stand behind patient
4)   Palpate the thyroid including the lobes and the isthmus


## PALPATION

Head
What do the masses feel like (hard, soft, variable, fluctuant)?
Are they mobile? Are they symmetrical? What are the borders like?
Is the fontanelle normally sized, large or small? Is it flat, sunken or bulging?
Are the sutures symmetric? Are they flat or prominent?

Neck
Is the neck supple?
Evaluate masses as in the head for location (midline, lateral) and quality as above
Are midline structures in the midline?
See technique for thyroid examination above

# PERCUSSION

Head:
   Is the skull tympanitic (cracked-pot sound)?

## Auscultation

   Head and Neck:
   Are there bruits?
   Listen for breath sounds in the neck (loudness, quality)

# EYE EXAMINATION

## Observation

### Extraocular movements
Are the eyes positioned in the midline? Are they always there or does the position vary? Does the ophthalmoscope light reflect in the midline (Hirschberg test)?
   Perform the "cover/uncover test" as indicated

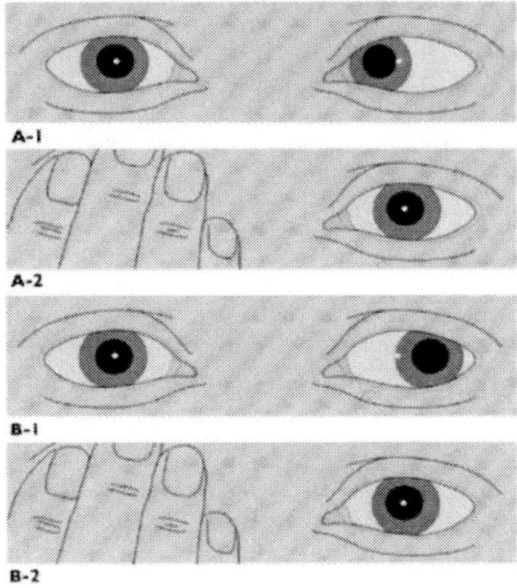

The Cover/Uncover test.

Do the eyes move in a conjugate manner? (Follow finger around)

Are there spontaneous movements not in patient's control? Are they horizontal, vertical or random?

Globe

Size

Enophthalmos

Exophthalmos

Lids

Is the lid position normal?

Are there any lesions or discolorations?

Are there any spontaneous movements?

Are there any lesions or foreign bodies on the inner lid, Evert the lids.

Canthi

Swelling or discoloration

Tearing (normal, wet or dry)

Exudates

Folds

Distance between inner canthi (hypo/hyper telorism)

Sclerae

Color of sclera (white, red, blue, yellow)

Exudates

Lesions or pigmentation on sclera including foreign bodies

Conjunctivae (both scleral and bulbar)

Color, uniformity (even redness, hemorrhages)

Swelling (edema, chemosis)

Lesions of foreign bodies (direct observation, blue light or fluorescein dye exam)

Corneas

Size

Color

Clarity (haziness, whiteness, presence of blood)

Lesions or foreign objects (direct observation or fluorescein dye)

Pupils

Size and state and equality of dilation

Roundness (if misshapen, describe how)

Response to light

Accommodation

Fundi
Optic disk for sharpness and color
Optic cup for size
Diameter of vessels, AV-nicking and venous pulsations
Hemorrhages or exudates
Tests for visual acuity
Opticokinetic nystagmus
Snellen charts
Pictures
Tumbling E
Letters


## Palpation

Palpate any masses
Intra-ocular tension


## EARS, NOSE MOUTH AND THROAT EXAMINATION

## Ears

### *Observation*
Pinna: For formation (size, setting, rotation, shape of helix, anti helix, tragus, anti tragus)
For extraneous lesions (pits, tags)
Ear canal:
For patency
For color (clear, red)
For cerumen
For exudates and lesions
For lesions and foreign bodies
Tympanic membrane
For appearance (translucent, opaque, red)
For landmarks (light reflex, malleolus, umbo, pars tensa, pars flaccid)
For position (retracted, neutral, bulging)
For mobility (a MUST, using pneumatic otoscopy, must be able to demonstrate correct usage of pneumatic otoscope)

Tricks of the trade - Obtain proper seal using a large enough speculum. There should be resistance in the ear canal if there is a tight seal. If ear drum appears retracted, assess for motion by observing most closely when providing negative pressure with the bulb. If there is motion, the eardrum is not glued down. If a patient is resisting (crying, Valsalva maneuver), squeeze the bulb very rapidly and observe most closely for motion during inhalation of the patient. This will be the time of least opposing pressure in the middle ear and will allow for detection of eardrum motion.

    For drainage, perforation
    Ancillary testing and interpretation
    Audiometry
    Tympanometry


# Nose

### *Observation*
External
    Size, shape and symmetry of nose and septum
    Are there signs of obstruction, unilateral or bilateral?

Trick of the trade - Have patient breathe out on tissue paper dangled in front of nose with and without manual obstruction of each nostril. If there is free flow of air unilaterally, then blockage is distal to the bifurcation at the nasal airway. If free flow unilaterally or bilaterally, there is no obstruction proximal to the bifurcation.

    Coloration
    Discharges (clear, cloudy, purulent), unilateral, bilateral?
    Odors
    Sounds (indicating possible obstruction)
    Internal
    Mucosa: Color, swelling?
    Turbinates: Color, swelling?
    Septum: Straightness, any visible masses?
    Foreign objects

### *Palpation*
Masses, external or internal for size, shape, color, mobility

Sinus tenderness

***Percussion***
Sinus tenderness


## Mouth and throat

***Observation (visual, olfactory)***
Lips: color, hydration, lesions
  Gums: color, lesions
  Buccal mucosa: color, lesions
  Teeth: Number formation, state of enamel
  Tongue: color, lesions, nature of papillae. Check upper and lower frenulum
  Palate: intactness (visual), uvula, formation, position (straight or deviated), soft palate (symmetry, lesions)
  Pharynx: color, lesions (tonsillar pillars, posterior wall of pharynx), odors
  Tonsils: redness, exudates, symmetry, lesions

***Palpation***
Check palate for intactness to palpation
  Palpate any lesions for fluctuance and tenderness


## Thorax examination

Tricks of the trade for performing respiratory examination on infants and children:
  Use a warm well-lit room with a minimum of distraction.
  Do as much of the exam as possible with child on parent's lap
  Use warm instruments!
  Quiet breathing is best heard during sucking or feeding.
  Lung sounds are best heard during inspiratory phase in a crying infant or toddler
  Guard privacy of adolescents with proper draping and gowns; perform exam without parents present.
  The passive exam is always best, e. g. decubitus position, supine position or during sleep.

## Chest wall

### *Observation*
Check for symmetry, deformities, and lesions, hypo- or hyper expansion.

Check respiratory rate, quality regularity and depth. Is there distress? Is there use of accessory muscles of respiration? Is chest expansion and retraction consistent with inhalation and exhalation (paradoxical breathing)?

Breast exam:

Tanner staging

Observe for symmetry, malformations, variability in size and shape, gynecomastia in males

Nipple: number, location, size, discharge?

### *Palpation*
Palpate for masses, irregularities, malformations

Palpate for tenderness to locate pain or injury

Squeeze thorax from behind patient to evaluate for pain and tenderness

Hooking maneuver under costal margin to elicit pain

Breast exam: masses, location, borders, firm, cystic, induration, tenderness, mobility

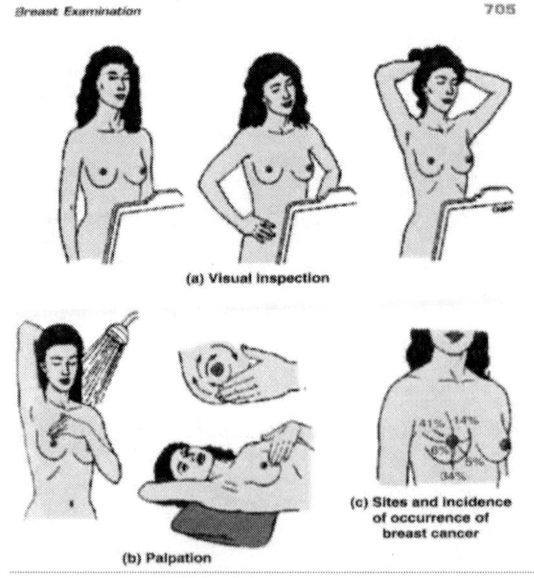


The breast examination.

## Pulmonary

### *Observation*
Observe as in "chest wall" above
> Breath: (sweet, fetid, acetone, etc)
> Color of patient (ruddy, cyanotic)
> Digital clubbing

### *Palpation*
Airway vibrations: Is there palpable fremitus?
> Palpate trachea for possible deviation
> Palpate to evaluate expansibility

### *Percussion*
Dullness vs. hyper-resonance
Note locations of both

### *Auscultation*
Identify entire respiratory cycle and place respiratory sounds in the cycle appropriately.
> Identify stridor on inhalation
> Note inspiratory to expiratory ratio
> Is the patient grunting with each respiration?

Tricks of the trade – ideally auscultate when patient is calm and cooperative. If not possible, inhalation phase will reveal more information. If patient is cooperative, have him/her breathe deeply and exhale as fast as possible. This may elicit more noticeable prolonged expiration or possibly a wheeze.

### Characteristics of lung sounds

| Lung sound | Name | Location |
|---|---|---|
| Discontinuous fine, high-pitch, low amplitude, short duration | Fine crackles | Small to medium airways |
| Discontinuous coarse low pitch, high amplitude, long duration | Coarse crackles | Larger airways |
| Continuous high pitched | Wheezes | Central and lower airways |
| Continuous low pitched | Rhonchi | Larger airways |

**(Continued)**

| Lung sound | Name | Location |
|---|---|---|
| Continuous or discontinuous dry crackles heard peripherally | Pleural rub | Pleural space |
| Continuous or discontinuous musical high pitch sound over midline or neck | Stridor | Large airways and larynx |

Characteristics of cough
Is it dry or wet?
Does it sound barky? Honking?
Is it paroxysmal? Is it staccato-like? Is there a whoop?


# Cardiac

### *Observation*
Overall growth
    Alertness
    Respiratory patterns
    Fatigue
    Color (pallor, cyanosis, clubbing)
    Edema (peripheral), ascites (abdominal distention and fluid wave)
    Dysmorphic features that may be associated with congenital heart disease

### *Palpation*
PMI (point of maximal intensity)
    Palpable thrills, heaves
    Pulses (rate, regularity, intensity, location, presence or absence, timing comparing upper to lower extremities)
    Liver size
    Peripheral edema

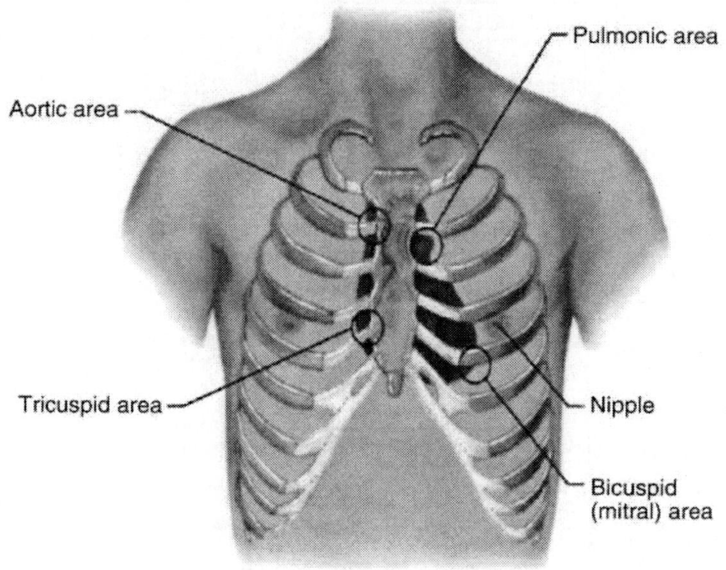

Cardiac Valve Areas for Precordial Auscultation. (*From Van de Graaff KH:* Human Anatomy. *New York: McGraw-Hill,* 2002, *Fig. 16.13, p. 554).*

### *Percussion*
Cardiac size (older children, adolescents)
    Dullness to percussion (fluid accumulation)
    Liver size
    **Auscultation** Tips: Listen first if a child is calm (carpe diem), do whatever it takes to distract a child
    Location of valve areas
    Heart tones ($S_1$, $S_2$)
    Relation to cardiac cycle
    Intensity of sounds
    Splitting of sounds
    Variation (or lack) of split sounds and heart rate with respiration, position, Valsalva maneuver
    Incidental sounds
    Gallops ($S_3$, $S_4$)
    Rubs (squeaky sounds, association with heartbeats)
    Clicks (timing in systole, early, mid, late (EML))
    Murmurs
    Timing in cardiac cycle, systolic (EML), diastolic (EML), holosystolic

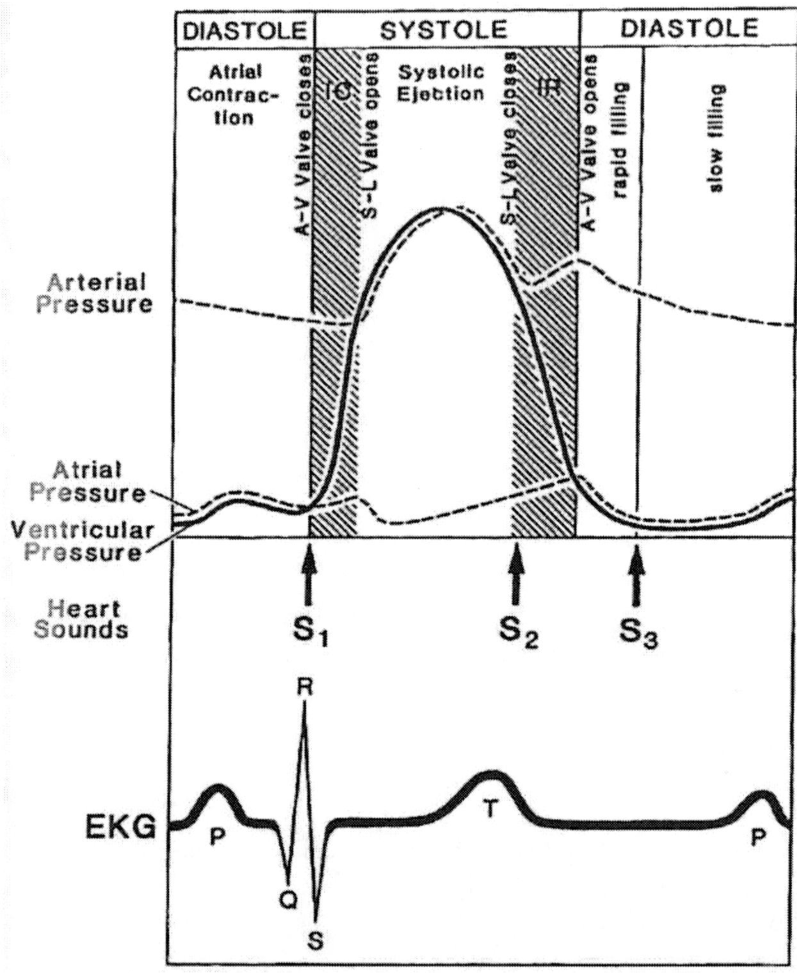



The Cardiac Cycle. (After CJ Wiggers: Nelson Textbook of Pediatrics, 17th ed. 2004, Fig. 413-3, p. 1488).

Intensity (Grade I-VI for systolic, Grade I-IV for diastolic)
Quality: musical, harsh, ejection (blowing, crescendo-decrescendo)
Location of intensity (relation of sternum, valve areas, base apex)
Variation with position (upright, recumbent, head straight or turned)

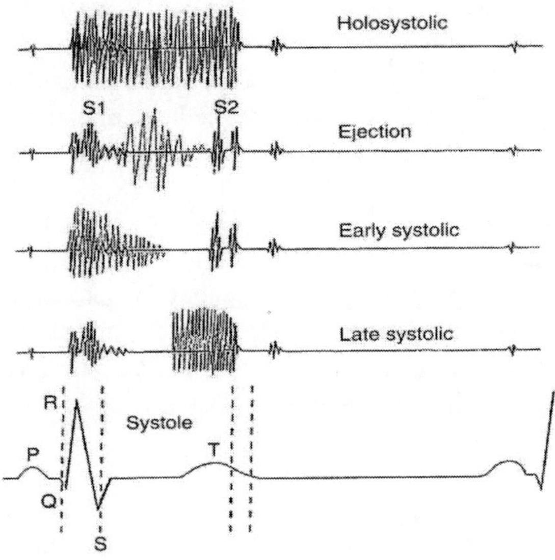


Systolic Murmur Classification.

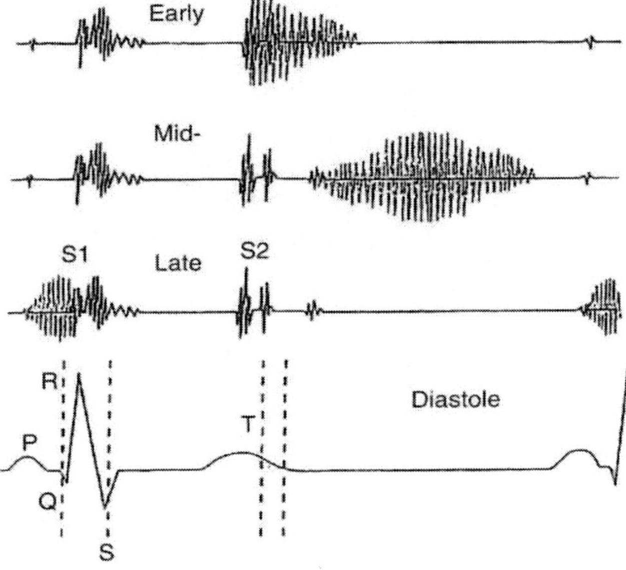


Diastolic Murmur Classification.

# ABDOMINAL, INGUINAL, ANAL AND RECTAL EXAMINATION

## Abdomen
Tricks of the trade – Do your best to distract the patient during the exam with any conversation you can muster. Use the head of a stethoscope to assess for tenderness. These will help if the patient is edgy or ticklish.

### *Observation*
Abdominal regions

Abdominal Shape: Round, flat, scaphoid. Is there distention?

Skin of abdomen: Taut, loose (indicative of nutritional status), peristaltic waves, visible bleeding (bruising, petechiae, purpura), visible blood vessels, jaundice (orange-yellow vs. greenish yellow)

### *Palpation*
Is it soft or hard?

Is there any tenderness? Locate tenderness (quadrants, midline, abdominal wall or deeper, flank) Does the pain radiate during pressure on the abdomen? Use directional palpation.

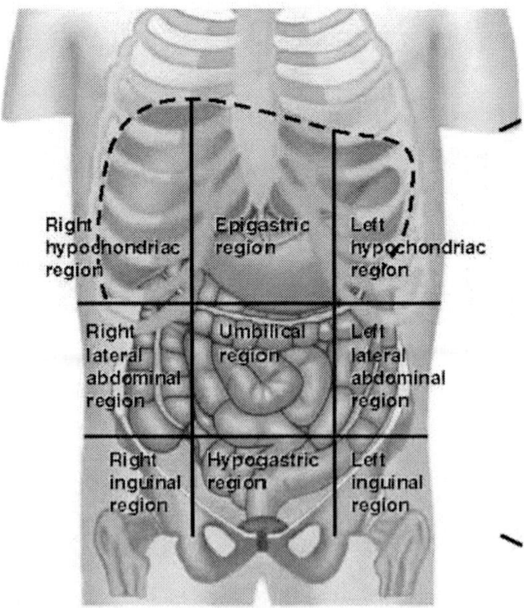


The abdominal regions.

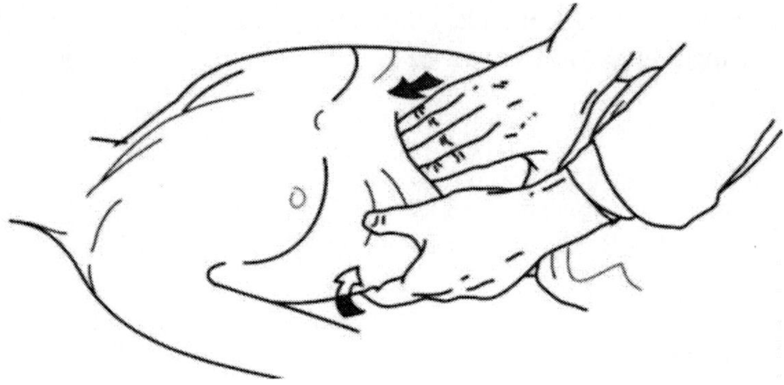

Palpating abdominal quadrants.

Is there guarding? Is it voluntary or involuntary? Is there rebound tenderness?

Check for psoas and obturator signs to assess peritoneal irritation. Also have patient jump of floor, if possible.

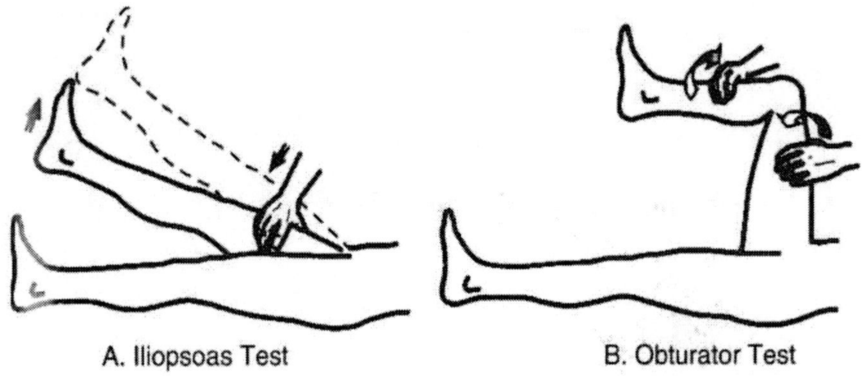



Check signs for ascites (peritoneal fluid wave).

Are there masses? Locate them. Are they soft, firm? Are they mobile? Are they tender or non-tender? Include inguinal area in the evaluation.

Hernia examination

- Have patient stand
- Inspect and palpate inguinal and femoral areas as patient performs Valsalva maneuver

- Palpate external inguinal ring alongside of scrotum, bilaterally; have patient either bear down or cough while inserting finger in inguinal ring.

### *Percussion*
Is it tympanitic? (Excess gas)
Dullness (over liver and spleen to determine size)

### *Auscultation*
Bowel sounds

Tricks of the trade: always listen before vigorous palpation; listen first if a child is calm, because this might not last too long
Presence (hypo- or hyperactive, pitch, localization)
Absence

## Anal

### *Observation*
Check for presence, dimple, patency, fissures, masses (size and color), fistulous tracts nearby. Check surrounding skin for color, erosions

## Rectal

### *Observation*
Check stool obtained for amount and color

### *Palpation*
Trick of the trade: explain whole procedure to patient and talk him/her through it. If a child, have parent there to help reassure and distract
Patency, tone, tenderness (local as well as abdominal on insertion)

# GENITALIA EXAMINATION

## Male

### *Observation*

*Gestalt* Is there any question of ambiguity?

Penis: Check for size, malformations, rotation, straightness, openings (extras), and signs of trauma or body art. Do Tanner staging. Are there any discharges? Check foreskin for presence, absence.

Testes: Size, shape, tenderness, color, descent, retractable, scrotal masses (testicular or extra-testicular), Tanner Staging. Use transillumination to determine solid mass from fluid collection.

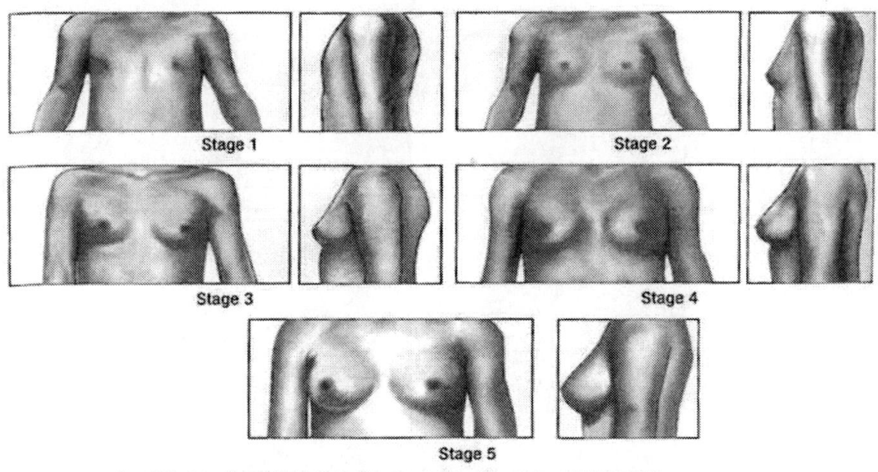


Tanner staging of breasts.

### *Palpation*

Penis: Check foreskin, if present, for retraction

Scrotal masses (testicular or extra-testicular) Do they feel hard, soft, like a bag of worms? Are they painful or tender? How does motion and location affect the pain?

Size and Tanner staging

## Female

### *Observation*

**Gestalt:** is there any question of ambiguity or masculinization?
**Vulva:** (mons pubis, clitoris, labia majora, labia minora). Check for size, shape, prominence, signs of trauma, adhesions. Vagina includes hymen, vaginal orifice, vaginal vault and posterior fourchette. Check for size, malformations and signs of trauma. Check for signs of bleeding or discharge, irritation. Check for patency of vagina

### *Palpation*
Check for masses (size shape color, location, tenderness)

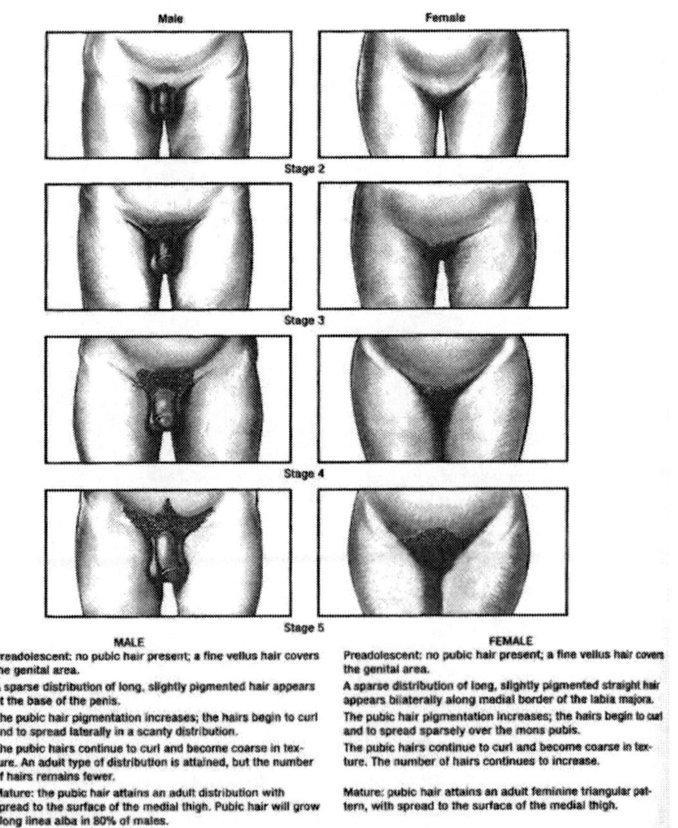


Tanner staging of genitalia.

# THE PELVIC EXAMINATION

## External exam

**Inspection** external genitalia (see above)
>**Palpation** Check for tenderness, masses of Bartholin glands.

### *Vaginal speculum exam*
Use a clean warmed speculum
>Insert initially at a 30° angle and then rotate until shorter blade is facing upward (90° angle)
>Separate the blades
>Observe vaginal mucosa for redness, erosions, discharge
>Observe cervix for redness, erosions, discharge
>Collect specimens as needed for Pap smears or cultures
>Slowly withdraw speculum in reverse order or insertion

### *Bimanual pelvic exam*
Insert well-lubricated index and middle fingers into the vaginal cavity
>Use other hand for palpation
>Examine Bartholin glands and urethra by spreading labia with palpating hand
>Palpate bladder and uterus by placing palpating hand over the inserted hand. The bladder is best felt by the inserted hand and the uterus by the palpating hand
>Palpate adnexae for ovarian size, fallopian tube size and masses or tenderness by placing inserted fingers lateral to the cervix and meeting the fingers with the examining hand compressing from above.

### *Rectovaginal exam*
This allows for better palpation of uterine placement, masses, ligaments and cul-de-sac.


## Extremities (non musculoskeletal) examination

### *Observation*
Malformations
>Swelling (diffuse or localized)

Cyanosis or clubbing
Signs of trauma

**Palpation**
Similar to observation above


# Musculoskeletal examination – general

**Observation**
Gait and posture – straightness of spine, symmetry or asymmetry of gait, favoring one side (antalgic gait), width or narrowness of base of gait, gluteal weakness (Trendelenburg gait), distal muscle weakness (steppage gait)

Head – Check for size, shape, signs of trauma

Neck – Swelling, deformity, masses, range of motion, tone, spinal curvature

Shoulders – Check for position of scapula, scapulo-humeral rhythm, winging of scapula, position of acromio-clavicular (AC) joint

Upper limbs – symmetry, atrophy or hypertrophy, positioning, joint swelling, malformations, range of motion

Lower limbs – see upper limbs above. Measure hip rotation angle and thigh-foot angle. Know normal progression of thigh-foot angle. Measure the leg length from the anterior superior iliac crest to the medial malleolus. Check for genu varum or valgum.

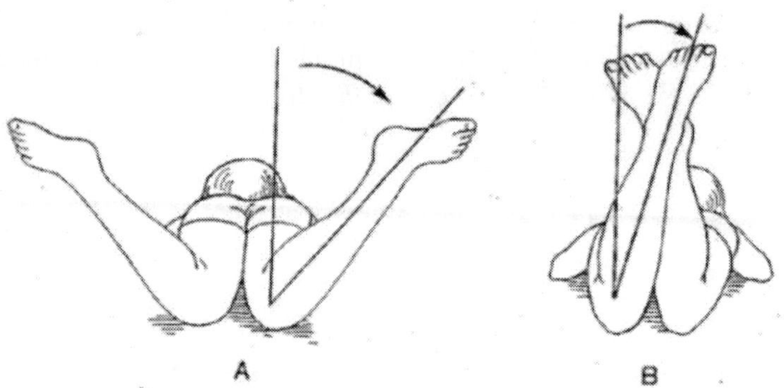


Hip Rotation measurement.

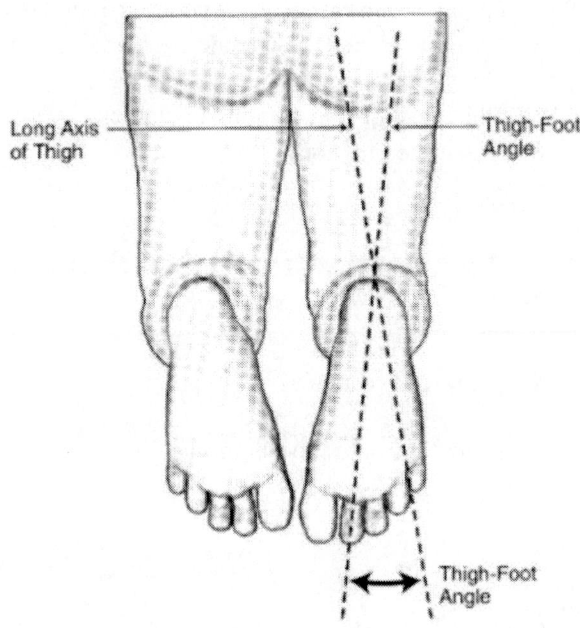


Thigh-foot angle measurement.

Spine – check for straightness or curvature in upright and flexed positions, positioning of pelvis, adventitial findings such as tufts of hair, pits or swelling in midline

Hips and groin – check for range of motion, flexibility and dislocation (Barlow and Ortolani tests)

### *Palpation*

Gait and posture – palpate muscles for hypertrophy or atrophy

Head – Palpate any masses or malformations of sutures or scalp swellings for location, induration, and tenderness.

Neck - Check for strength and tone, range of motion, tenderness. Evaluate masses for size, location, induration, mobility and tenderness.

Upper limbs – Check for strength and tone. Palpate from mid-clavicle to hand for range of motion, pain and tenderness and for joint swelling and effusion. Evaluate masses for size, location, induration, mobility and tenderness.

Lower limbs – Palpate from the anterior superior iliac crest to the bottom of feet; check range of motion, pain and tenderness and for joint swelling and effusion.

Spine – Palpate for bony or paraspinous tenderness. Test muscle strength of back muscles in the supine position.


## MUSCULOSKELETAL EXAMINATION – SPORTS MEDICINE SPECIAL TESTS

### Shoulders and upper extremities

Neer test - Fast forward flexion of the humerus will elicit pain. Tests rotator cuff

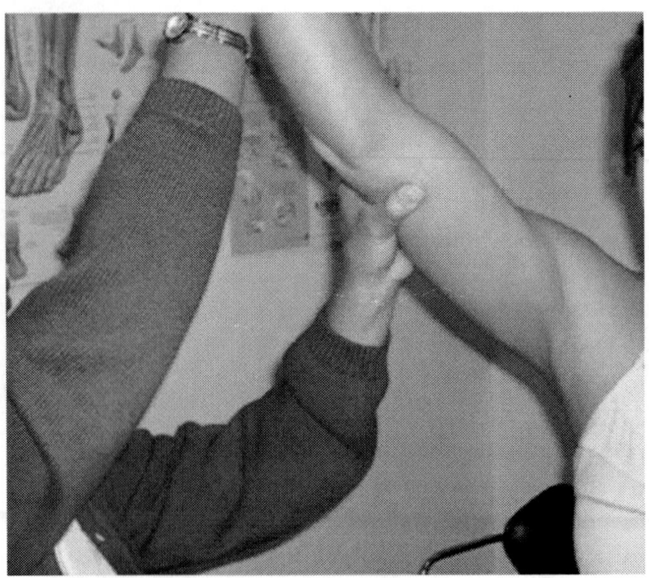

Neer test.

Hawkins-Kennedy test – Internal rotation of the humerus with abduction and forward flexion of the humerus will produce pain. Test for rotator cuff impingement

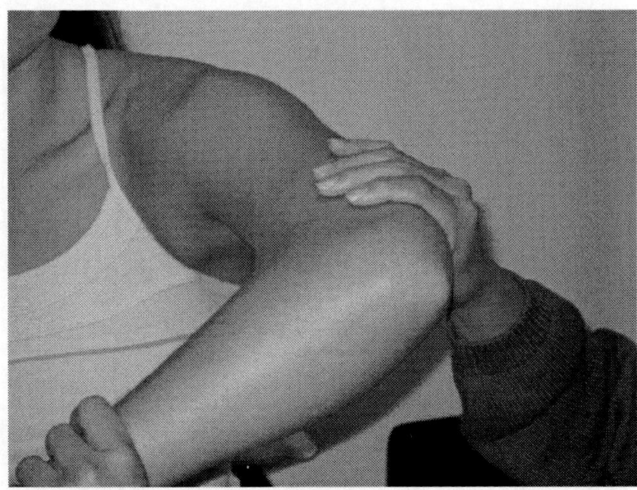

Hawkins-Kennedy test.

Jobe relocation test – with patient supine hang arm off the edge of the table with shoulder abducted 90°, externally rotate the humerus. This will cause discomfort. With hand on shoulder pushing posterior, the discomfort will be relieved. This tests for anterior instability of shoulder.

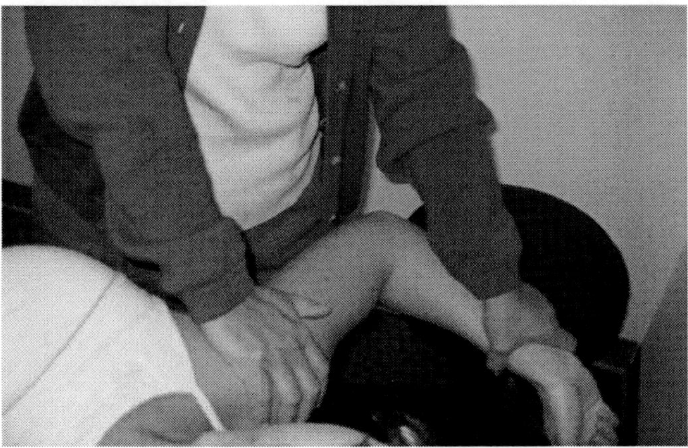

Jobe test.

Load-and-shift test – Grasp shoulder with patient's arm held downward with elbow flexed at 90°. With other hand, the examiner will move the shoulder joint in all directions to test for laxity.

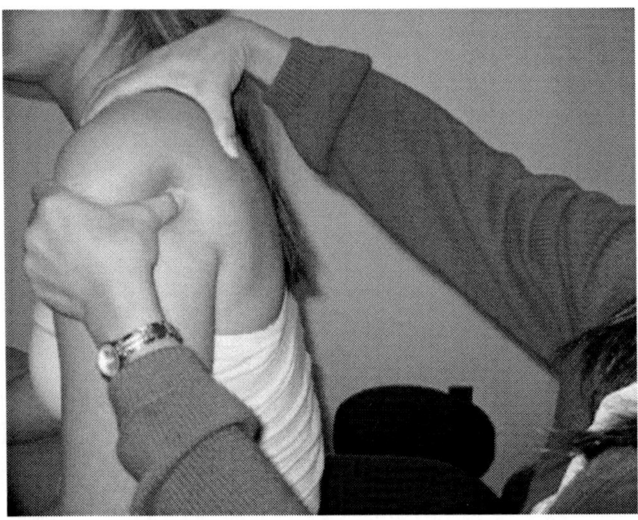

Load and shift test.

Supraspinatus (empty can) test – With arm abducted 90°, forward flexed at 30° and internally rotated (thumbs-down position) check for weakness or pain on movement by having patient pull up arm against resistance from the examiner.

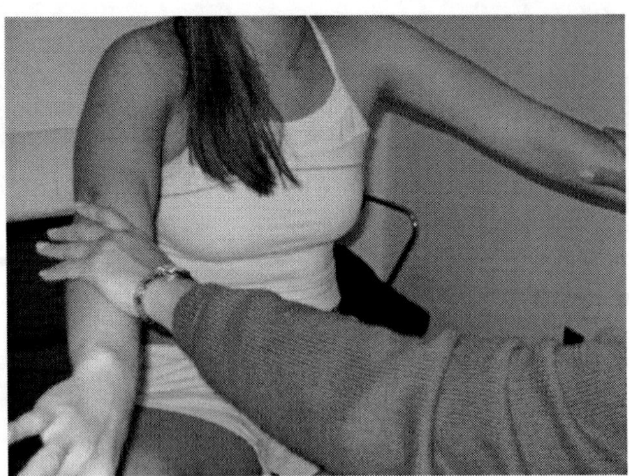

Supraspinatus test.

Cross adduction test – Adduct arm 90° across chest to assess AC joint.

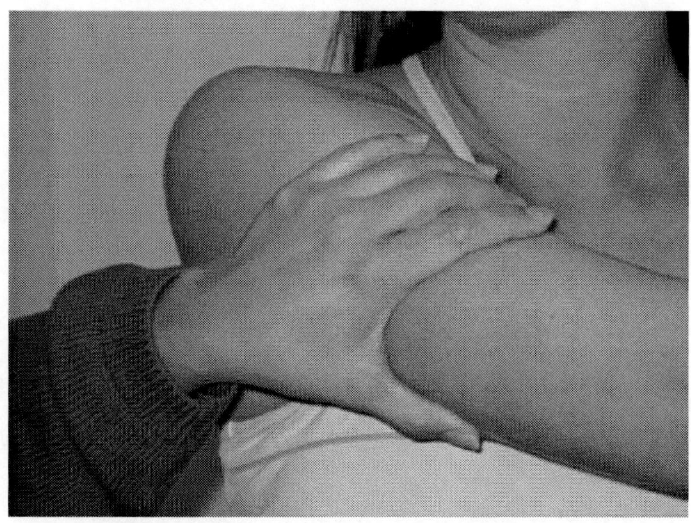

Cross adduction test.

Speed test – Opposite of empty can test (thumbs up). Tests long head of biceps

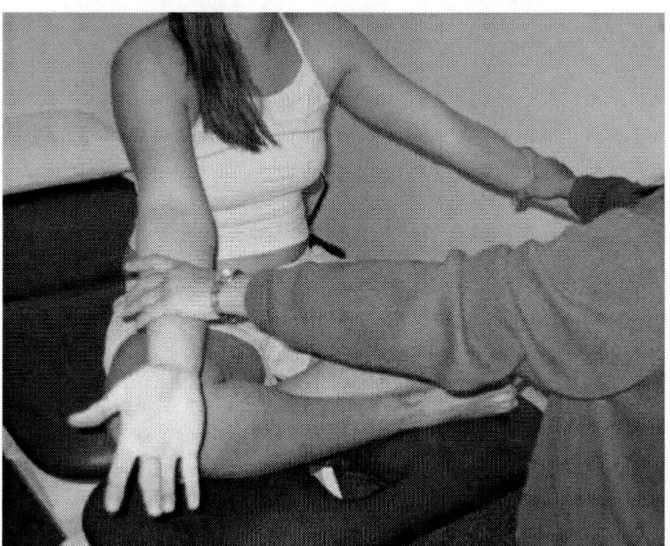

Speed test.

Check for swelling, range of motion of elbow, wrist and finger joints

## SPINE AND BACK

## Standing

Check for curvature upright and with bending (Adams test).

Hyperextension test - Have patient stand on one leg and hyperextend back. Does this elicit pain?

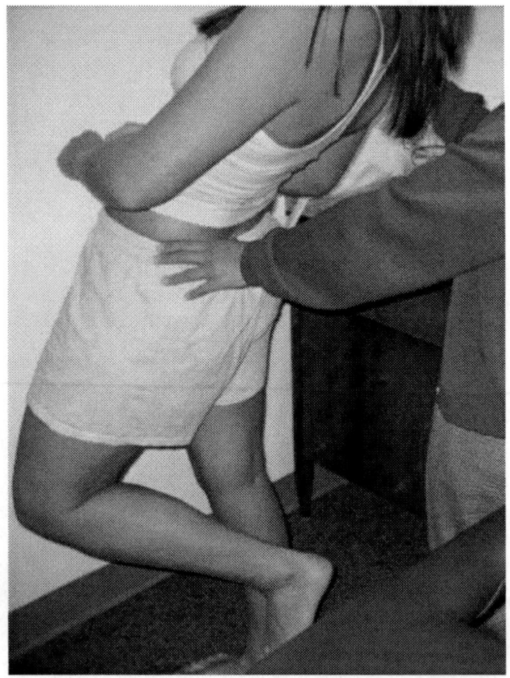

Hyperextension test.

Trendelenburg test – In hyperextension of back, patient's gluteus muscle will sag on the weak side.

Test calf muscle strength by repeated heel raises by standing on one leg and bending the knee of the other leg.

Test anterior tibialis strength by heel-walking

Supine

Raising an extended let will elicit sciatic pain

Flex, abduct and externally rotate leg ("4" position) to test for sacroiliac pain (Faber or Patrick test)

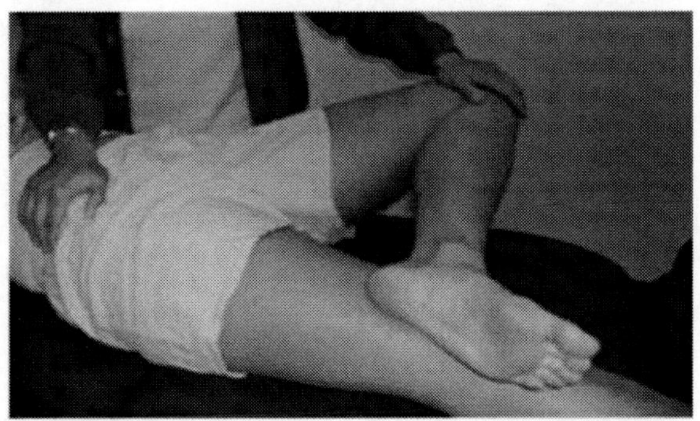

Patrick test.

Prone
Hyperextend back - Postural kyphosis will correct itself, pathologic kyphosis will not.

## LOWER EXTREMITIES

## Knee

Patellar apprehension test – With patient supine and knee slightly flexed apply laterally directed force to the patella.

Lachman test – With patient supine on table and knees at 30°, stabilize the femur with one hand above the knee. Move the tibia/fibula anterior-posterior with the other hand (tests anterior cruciate ligament).

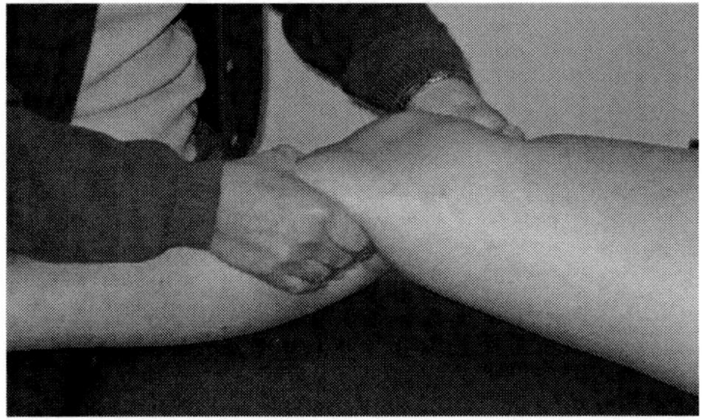

Lachman test.

McMurray test –Hold one hand on the knee and hold the foot with the other hand with knee at about 45° with patient supine on the table. Then extend knee while rotating it either medially or laterally (tests menisci).

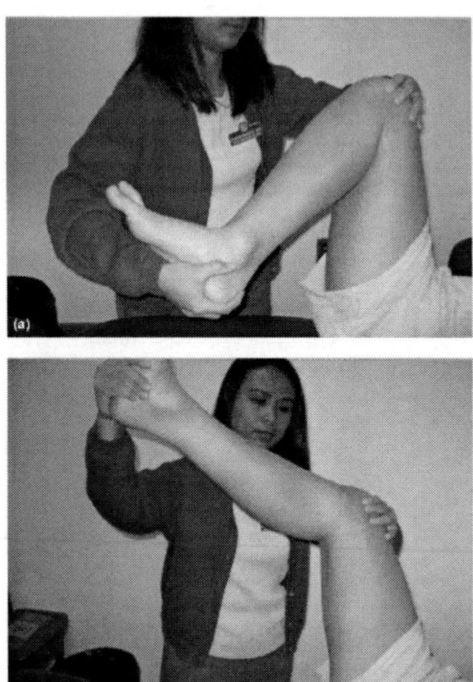

McMurray test.

Varus and valgus stress tests – With one hand holding the thigh above the knee and the other hand holding the shin below the knee apply alternating valgus and varus stress to the knee joint (tests medial and collateral ligaments).


## Ankle

Anterior drawer test – Hold distal shin with one hand and grab the heel with the other. Move foot forward and backward (tests anterior talo-fibular ligament)

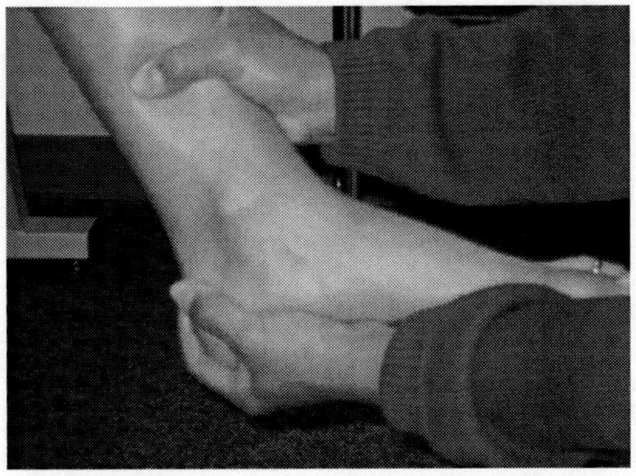

Anterior drawer test for ankle.

Talar tilt – Holding foot as above do an inversion maneuver of the foot (tests calcaneo-fibular ligament)

External rotation test – similarly, rotate the foot externally (tests tibiofibular syndesmosis)

Squeeze test – Holding the knee at 90° squeeze the distal calf (tests tibio-fibular syndesmosis)

## NEUROLOGIC EXAMINATION

### Gestalt

Note facies and check for dysmorphic features
    Check for obvious abnormalities in head size and shape
    Check for tone and posture
    Assess overall developmental level (first impression)
    Any obvious odors (musty, sweet, sour)

### Meningeal – signs of irritation

Kernig sign – with patient supine, flex leg to 90°. Then straighten knee. This will elicit pain and discomfort.

Brudzinski sign – with patient supine, flex neck. This will feel stiff and will elicit pain and discomfort.

## Cerebral – higher cognitive functioning

***Observation***
Check skull for size and shape. Do an actual measurement and plot on growth chart

# MINI MENTAL STATUS EXAM

- Orientation (x3, self, time and place)
- Registration (Name three objects and ask patient to repeat them until they are learned. Record the number of trials).
- Attention and Calculation (Subtracting serial 7s)
- Recall (Ask patient to recall the 3 objects learned in "registration" above
- Language (Name objects, 3-stage commands, reading, writing, copying geometric figures)

***Palpation***
Palpate skull for fontanel size and shape, sutures for patency or closure, masses, signs of trauma

***Percussion***
"Cracked-pot" sound for fluid

***Auscultation***
Listen for bruits

## Cerebellar – assess balance and coordination

***Observation***
Stationary testing (Romberg sign) - Stand patient upright and check ability to maintain balance with eyes closed

Gait examination - Wavering, lurching, festinating, and ataxic gait (is it due to weakness or poor coordination?) Differentiate coordination by performing heel-to-shin maneuver with patient recumbent to factor out gravity and weakness.

Diadochokinesia – this is the ability to substitute quickly a motor impulse with an opposing one (rapid alternating movements. Assess the patient's ability to avoid hitting self when examiner releases patient's hand that is aimed towards self.

Dyssynergia – impairment of voluntary movements (fractionated or jerky)

Dysmetria – ability to judge distances with voluntary movement (finger-to nose)

Fine motor skills – includes tremors

Head titubation

Labyrinthine tests: to rule out cerebellar problem – nystagmus. Check for direction, fast and slow component.


## Brain stem – assess cranial nerve function

Olfactory I: Identify substance with a known odor (coffee) with eyes closed

Ophthalmic II: Careful fundoscopic exam to assess for sharpness or optic disk, optic cup size, engorgement of blood vessels, venous pulsations. Assess visual fields.

Oculomotor III, trochlear IV and abducent VI: lateral gaze VI, downward medial gaze IV, all other movement, III.

Trigeminal V: Sensory to face, ophthalmic, maxillary and mandibular branches.

Motor: chewing (temporalis and masseter muscles). Observe motor function by symmetry and strength of bite and by palpating muscle mass.

Facial VII: Sensory: taste, anterior 2/3 of tongue

Autonomic: salivary gland secretion

Motor: muscles of facial expression, stapedius, stylohyoid and digastric muscles. Check for eye droop, nasolabial fold fullness, raising and closing of eyes, showing teeth, natural smile and puffing of cheeks.

Auditory VIII: Tuning fork for high, mid and low frequency losses. Comare hearing with fork on skull bones with fork in front of ear (air conduction vs. bone conduction) Conductive hearing loss will have a difference, sensorineural loss will not (air-bone gap).

Glossopharyngeal IX. Taste posterior third of tongue, sensation in pharynx

Vagus X: Supplies palate and pharynx (similar to IX), and motor fibers to neck, thorax and abdomen. Check for gag reflex, asymmetry of palate and hoarseness.

Accessory XI: Strength of trapezius and sternocleidomastoid muscles. Have patient shrug shoulders and move head laterally against resistance.

Hypoglossal XII: Motor nerve of tongue. Check for movement and symmetry.


## Spinal reflexes – assess reflex arc at all spinal levels

### *Observation/percussion*

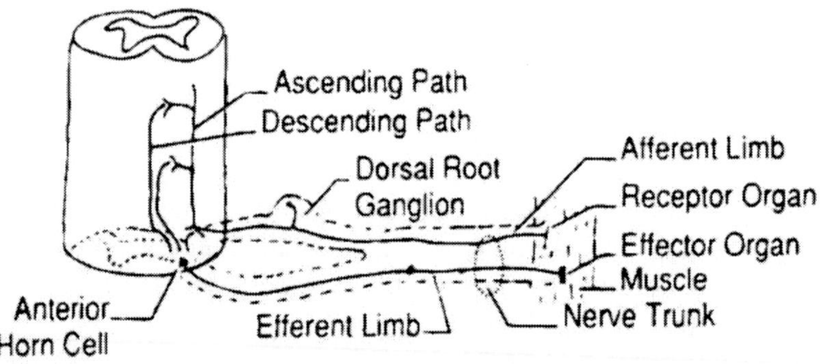


The reflex arc.


**Measuring reflex responses**

> 0 – no response
> 1+ Detectable, but weak
> 2+Easliy detectable
> 3+Brisk with at most a few beats of clonus
> 4+Sustained clonus
> Trick of the trade – if reflexes are absent or 1+ have patient curl fingers of both hands tightly, interlock them in front of chest and pull hands apart against resistance of the fingers. This may help elicit a stronger response when tapping the tendon.

# Sensory

## *Palpation*

Test for light touch, deep pain, pinprick, heat, cold, position sense (proprioception – toe up or down), stereogenesis (feeling familiar objects with eyes closed) two-point discrimination (ability to feel two needles at the same time – move them closer until the patient can no longer discriminate) and vibratory sense (tuning fork)

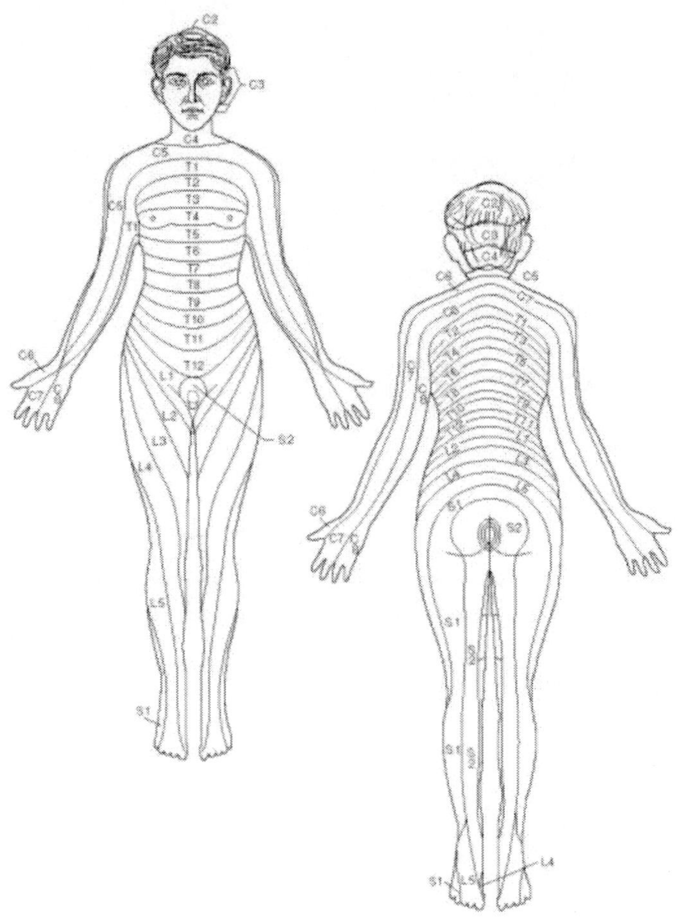

Point-by point sensory representation – dermatomes.

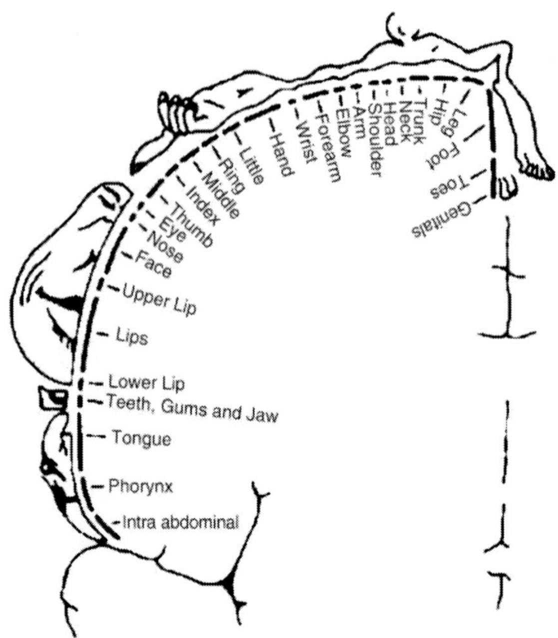


Point-by-point sensory representation – cerebral.


## Motor

### *Observation*

Evaluate for muscle hypertrophy or atrophy

Does patient climb up thigh when trying to stand? (Gower sign for proximal weakness)

Gait – ataxic, antalgic, steppage, Trendelenburg

Tricks of the trade – Consider a non-neurologic cause of ataxia if patient has extremely awkward/lurching gait, but never falls. Remember - It requires greater strength and coordination not to fall when in a bizarre anti-gravity position. Also, have patient lie recumbent and cradle both heels in your hands while keeping your hands on the table. Ask patient to raise one leg. Normally, the other heel will press down on your cradling hand. (Hoover sign).


### *Palpation*

Check for atrophy, hypertrophy, tone and tenderness.

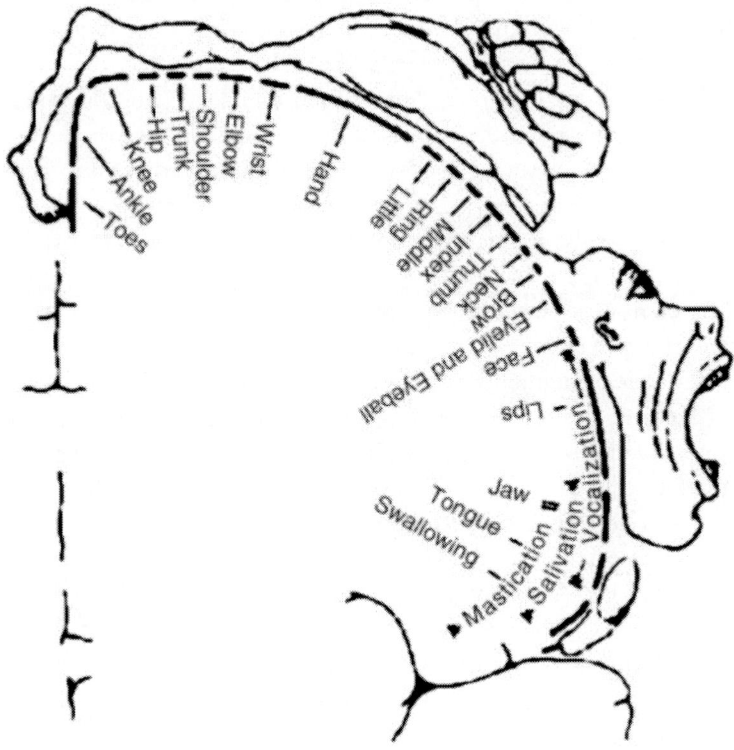


Point-by-point representation of motor areas in the parietal lobe.

## Dermatologic examination

### *Observation and palpation*

### Configuration
Macules – flat circumscribed lesions, visible to the eye and not palpable. However, still palpate them for tenderness and color change

Papules – raised lesions ≤ 1cm in diameter. They are non-mobile and extend to the surface of the dermis. Also, palpate these for tenderness and color change (erythema and edema as in **Darier's sign**). Scratch areas nearby to see if new lesions arise (**Koebner phenomenon**).

Plaques – Papules or collections of them >1cm. in diameter.

Pustules – Papules containing white blood cells and serum (pus).

Abscesses- these are larger collections of pus that run deeper into the subcutaneous tissue and the dermis. There may be associated sinus tracts connecting to the surface or to deeper internal structures.

Nodules – Elevated lesions, deeper than papules. They do not attach to overlying dermis; therefore the dermis is freely mobile above the lesion.

Cysts – sharply circumscribed movable nodules containing fluid (e. g. serum, pus, sebum)

Vesicles – sharply marginated superficial collections of clear fluid located in the epidermis ≤1 cm in diameter. Does palpation or scratching of normal skin nearby elicit new vesicles (**Nikolsky sign**)?

Bullae - Large vesicles > 1 cm in diameter

Scales - Dried fragments of dead skin. Does removal of a scale induce bleeding (**Auspitz' sign**)? May be secondary to infection or inflammation

Erosions - Scratch marks on the skin usually due to loss of epidermis due to rupture of a vesicle

Crusts – dried exudates from serum, pus, blood. There is an antecedent lesion such as a vesicle, pustule, abscess or erosion.

Lichenifications – extensive areas of dried plaques induced by repeated scratching

Ulcers – Depressed lesions with loss of both epidermis and dermis. They can be a consequence of infection, trauma, and malignancy. Palpate them for anesthesia or tenderness.

Induration/sclerosis – hardening of the skin characterized by thickening and often a result of previous infection or trauma.

Scars – these are due to formation of new connective tissue after destruction of the epidermis, dermis and subcutaneous tissue.

Fissures – these are painful cracks in the skin owing to inflammation.

Color

Red – increased blood flow or inflammation

Purple – increased venous blood flow or blood extravasation. Palpation of areas of increased blood flow will blanch, areas of extravasation will not.

Brown or black – indicates pigment deposit

Blue – pigment deposit or venous vascular collection

Green – pigment deposit or resolving hematoma

Yellow – contains fat or sebum

Flesh colored – lesion with normal overlying skin

White – depigmentation or keratin deposits

Pattern

Shape

Round
Oval
Linear or serpigenous
Amorphous
Definition
Regularity (Are lesions similar or variable at a given time?)
Uniformity (is there central clearing, is it spotty?)
Sharpness of border
Variability
Persistent
Evanescent
Distribution
Flexural
Dermatomal or lines of Blaschko (embryologic lines of development)
Polar
Areas of exposure or non-exposure
Unique patterns (condition-specific)

# Chapter 3

# MEDICAL REASONING: PUTTNG IT ALL TOGETHER

## BASIC OUTLINE

I.   The full data collection
   A. Day one of the first clinical clerkship, a tabula rasa
   B. Illustrative case (abbreviated, mercifully)
II.  Generating hypotheses - The narrowing process
   A. Classifying
      1.   Systemic
      2.   Etiologic
      3.   Physiologic
      4.   Epidemiologic
   B. Prioritizing
      1.   Prevalence
      2.   The time factor
III. Testing hypotheses
IV.  Re-testing hypotheses
V.   Heuristics
      1.   Pattern recognition
      2.   Augenblick
VI.  Pitfalls in diagnosis
VII. Overdiagnosis

VIII. Wisdom attained over the years: Summary of clinical aphorisms
learned from my preceptors and life including some hard knocks;
antidotes to mines in the field.


# EXPANSION OF BASIC OUTLINE

## The full data collection: Day 1 of the student clinical clerkship

(Curtain rises. Student and attending physician are in the preceptor room after
student has done a complete history and physical examination)


### *Medical student*
"Chief complaint:
Patient is a 6 year-old girl with a fever and a rash of three days duration.


### *History of present illness*
She is a previously healthy child with normal growth and development, well
until 3 days ago when she developed fever. There was pain in her throat about
6/10 exacerbated by swallowing. Solid food intake has been slightly less due
to the pain, but patient is taking fluids OK. The pain tends to get worse at
night. There is occasional headache. She vomited once and there is no
diarrhea, constipation or abdominal pain. There are no visual changes and no
history of redness of the eyes. Hearing is normal and there is no ear pain or
stuffiness. There is no nasal congestion, with no discharge or any itching or
pain. There is throat pain, but no obstruction to swallowing, no drooling. There
is no history of neck pain swelling or stiffness. No chest pain, coughing,
wheezing, stridor, dyspnea, tachypnea or apnea. There has been no change in
sensorium or thought processes, no balance problems or other forms of
incoordination. There are no sensory or motor abnormalities of the facial area
mouth or tongue. The rash appeared yesterday. It is not painful. There is no
history of trauma to the mouth or throat or any history of foreign body
ingestion. **(5 minutes have elapsed)**


### *Past history*
Medical: The patient is generally healthy. She has had 2 episodes of otitis
media in her life and has had no hospitalizations. She has had approximately
12 viral infections in her life. She has occasional functional constipation which
responds to Miralax.

Surgical: No injuries, no operations.

Allergies: No known food or drug allergies.

Medications: Miralax as mentioned above.

Immunizations: Up to date.

Safety precautions in the home and automobile were reviewed

Birth history: 40 week gestation, Caesarean section for breech position, mom was Group B strep positive. Mothers other serologies, rubella titer, RPR, HIV tests were all negative. Birth weight was 8# 9 oz and patient was in the hospital for 72 hours. She received Vitamin K, a Hepatitis B immunization and passed the state hearing screen. For the first three months, she was the fussiest baby ever known to mankind. **(5 more minutes have elapsed)**

### Family history

Father, age 39 alive and well (A&W). Mother, age 42 A&W. Dysplastic hip. Brother, age 4 A&W. Extensive family history presented including parents, grandparents and even some great-grandparents with all causes of death when remembered. **(7 more minutes have elapsed)**

### Personal and social history

Demographic: Patient is Caucasian female of British (English-Scottish) descent on her father's side and of Polish/Lithuanian/ Roumanian-German descent on her mother's side. The family's religion is Jewish and they are members of a Reform Congregation in town. She will be attending religious school next September and will also be starting 1st grade in public school.

Socioeconomic: Father is a househusband. Mother is a pediatric gastroenterologist. Father has a PhD degree and mother has an MD degree.

Life experiences: Patient loves to read and is learning this on her own with help from parents. She does ballet, gymnastics and is taking Suzuki cello lessons. She, along with her brother and two other first cousins are totally in love with their fatuous grandparents, as are their fatuous grandparents with them. There is no exposure to smoke and there is one dog in the home. There have been no travels except to amusement parks, water parks, trips to a camp somewhere in the middle of New Hampshire and occasional (not enough) visits to grandparents about 4 hours away." (10 more minutes have elapsed…are you getting the idea?)

Review of systems: (6 more minutes)

Developmental history (5 more minutes)

**Attending physician** (slapping himself to stay awake)
"And the physical examination…?"

*Medical student*
"Complete head-to-toe physical examination" **(15 minutes)**

**Attending physician:** "So, what do you think is going on?"

*Medical student*
Student presents a complete list of every condition that causes a fever, every condition that causes a sore throat (including gonorrhea and fish-bone embedded in tonsil) and every condition that causes vomiting. **(One hour, total time elapsed, 1 hour and 53 minutes)**

*Attending physician*
"So, what is **the** diagnosis?"

*Medical student*
"I dunno."

*Attending physician*
"Well, that's OK. This is first day of your first clerkship. Your presentation was very thorough and well-organized. Don't feel bad if you can't figure out the diagnosis, yet."

*Medical student*
"Does that mean you're not flunking me?"

*Attending physician*
"Yeah, no problem, let's go see the kid."

(Student and attending physician walk down the hall and knock on the exam room door)

**Attending physician** (standing at door):
"Hi, I'm Dr. Senior." (To patient): "Hi Ruthie, how're you doing." (To student): "This is scarlet fever." **(Time elapsed: 12 seconds)**

***Medical student***
"Wow, you're awesome. How'd you get it so fast?"

***Attending physician***
"I dunno. I guess I've been through so many of them; it's just part of me. Do you see how Ruthie has flushed cheeks and looks white about the mouth? I also noticed that her tongue looked kind of strawberry-ish. As soon as I opened the door there was an obvious odor of a bacterial infection in the room. It has been a long day and I appreciate everyone's patience, so since the clinical picture is so clear, we'll spare her a strep screen and just start her on a 10 day course of oral penicillin 250 mg tid. It will be fine for her to resume normal activities in 24 hours."

Dénouement: Ruthie was fine the next day and resumed her normal activities.

(Curtain falls to the tune of Verdi's Triumphal March from "Aida.")

## GENERATING HYPOTHESES – THE NARROWING PROCESS: THE THOUGHT PROCESS OF A RESIDENT WITH SOME EXPERIENCE

## Classifying

Our case discussion with the third year medical student on his first clerkship day was quite daunting. In the real world, a physician will have about 15 minutes in which to see this patient. So, how do we get from here to there in a lot less time? With experience and learning, a resident will acquire knowledge of how certain conditions present themselves. With this information at his/her fingertips, he/she will try to plug the facts into basic categories. The main frameworks we use are "systemic" and "etiologic." Therefore, if a certain symptom presents itself, the first question to ask is "To what system can we ascribe it?" For example, if a patient's chief complaint is leg pain, it might be reasonable to exclude the respiratory system, ears-nose-throat, etc. However, one must not be too quick to select only one system. Below is a table of conditions which may, at first, seem to come from only one system, but may also come from others.

| System | Problem | Other Causes |
| --- | --- | --- |
| GI | Jaundice | Heme: hemolytic anemia; metabolic: carotenemia |
| | Vomiting | CNS: ↑ICP, renal: uremia; endo: hypoadrenalism; ENT: labyrinthitis; psych: eating disorders |
| | Diarrhea | Endo: hyperthyroid, psychogenic |
| | Constipation | Endo: hypothyroid, psychogenic; CNS: cord lesions, CP; GU: UTI |
| | Abdominal pain | Pulm: pneumonia; GU: stones, UTI, PID, hematocolpos, hydronephrosis; endo: ↑$Ca^{2+}$, DKA, Addison's, psychogenic |
| | Hematemesis | Heme: bleeding diathesis; ENT: epistaxis |
| Pulmonary | Stridor | Endo: ↓$Ca^{2+}$; CNS: brain injury with vocal cord paralysis |
| | Cough | Cardiac: CHF; ENT: FB in ear; toxic: drug side effects; psychogenic: drug abuse ("huffing"), marijuana, habit cough, allergy; CNS: chronic aspiration |
| | Wheeze | Cardiac: CHF; endo: Addison's, allergy; GI: GERD; psych: vocal cord dysfunction |
| Pulmonary/ cardiac | Chest pain | Musculoskeletal: costochondritis, slipped rib; GI: pancreatitis, subphrenic abscess, GERD |
| | Cyanosis | Hepatogenic cyanosis; metabolic: methemoglobinemia; CNS: central hypoventilation, neuromuscular disease |
| | Tachypnea | Metabolic acidosis, psychogenic hyperventilation |
| | Hypertension | Renal disease (hyperaldosteronism); endo: hyperthyroid, Cushing's, hyperaldosteronism |
| | Hypotension | Endo: Addison's, hypothyroidism, congenital adrenal hyperplasia |
| | Bradycardia | Endo: hypothyroidism |
| | Tachycardia | Endo: hyperthyroidism; psych: anxiety |
| Renal/GU | Polyuria/freq | Endo: diabetes mellitus; CNS: central diabetes insipidus, spinal cord pathology, MS; psych: diuretic abuse, polydipsia, sexual abuse |
| | Oliguria/retention | Pulmonary and CNS: SIADH; CNS: spinal cord injury, demyelinating disease |
| | Hematuria | Hematol: bleeding diathesis, anticancer drugs; psych: factitious |
| CNS | Headache | Renal: hypertension; ENT: sinusitis, psychogenic |
| | Seizure | Metabolic: hypoglycemia, hyper/hypoelectrolytemias, hypocalcemia, inborn errors of metabolism; renal: uremia; psych: syncope, hyperventilation, narcolepsy; cardiac: arrhythmia; GI: GERD (Sandifer syndrome) |
| | Altered consciousness (lethargy, agitation) | Renal: uremia; hepatic: liver failure; endo: hypoadrenalism, DKA, hypoparathyroidism, hyperthyroidism; metabolic/toxic: Wilson disease, poisoning; pulmonary: $CO_2$ narcosis |
| | Focal weakness | Ortho: bone pain (Parrott's paralysis owing to injury, tumor, rickets, scurvy) |
| Psych | Psychosis | GI: Liver failure; GU: uremia; heme: porphyria lupus erythematosis; metab: Wilson disease |
| | Anxiety | Endo: hyperthyroidism, catecholamine excess, hypoparathyroidism; pulm: hypoxia; toxic: medications (steroids, catecholamines) |
| Endo | Poor linear growth | Renal, infectious, cardiac, pulmonary: chronic conditions of almost any kind |
| | Late puberty | GI: IBD; psych: eating disorders; CNS: craniopharyngioma; heme-onc: late effects of cancer treatment |

The next question to ask is "what is the etiology?" Typically, in pediatrics, etiologic classification is:

Congenital/genetic

Infectious/inflammatory

Nutritional/metabolic/toxic

Traumatic

Neoplastic

Vascular

Psychological

Thus, if a patient presents with a chief complaint of fever, one may think first of "infectious/inflammatory," but keep in mind, Neoplastic and vascular (vasculitis) are also possibilities, though more remote.

Further narrowing down may be based on epidemiology. For example, an X-linked recessive disorder rules out females (caveat, not always). Age is another factor. Certain conditions may be more prevalent in infants. Therefore if a patient is 19 years old, he will not have pyloric stenosis.

Winnow down more by looking at physiology. For example, if we have ascribed our diagnosis to the kidney, then we can decide of the condition is related to the glomeruli, tubules, etc. Or in the case of the lungs, consider large airways, small airways or alveoli. If a neurologic diagnosis is entertained, from where in the brain are the symptoms originating? Does abnormal liver function seem to be due to destruction or obstruction?

## Prioritizing

Making correct medical judgments can be difficult enough and this is compounded by the factor of time. The big question in the back of any clinician's mind should be "What do I want to know, and when do I want to know it?" One way of narrowing this down is prioritizing. Since "common things occur commonly", let's go with those conditions with higher prevalence. But the factor of time haunts us. Bacterial meningitis may be less common than a viral URI, but must be acted on right away. There is nary a physician who diagnoses bacterial meningitis who does not think or say: "I wish I could have done this tap sooner." Another aspect of prioritizing with time can be very helpful: the duration of the symptoms. Thus, if symptoms are of acute onset, or if ongoing for a year, they would shed different lights.

Another form of prioritizing is to review the constellation of symptoms, the groups you have developed and see if these symptoms appear in one or more of your groups.

## Where are we now?

Since the history comes first, the clinician will begin the sorting and eliminating process at that point. As in the scenario presented above, we have a 6 year old girl with a fever, sore throat and a rash with one episode of vomiting. That's all we know. So, when we generate a list of possibilities for diagnosis, it becomes slightly less overwhelming than Nelson's Textbook of Pediatrics in its entirety. Most of us, based on our life experience and even simple common sense have already eliminated several pages of Nelson, whether or not we are even conscious of it. We can pretty safely forget about congenital/genetic, nutritional/metabolic/toxic, traumatic, and psychogenic. But keep in the back of our minds that infectious/inflammatory conditions, malignancies and vasculitis, can cause fevers, sore throats and rashes.

The next sort is systemic. The constellation of symptoms could refer to the integumentary system (rash), immunologic system (sore throat, fever) and gastrointestinal system (vomiting, fever).

At this point, one may ask: "What about the headache?" "How do we know she doesn't have a brain tumor...or migraines? OK, add these diagnoses on, for now, but on a way back burner.

At this point, we can now generate our first differential diagnosis.


## Fever

Any infectious/inflammatory condition, bacterial, viral fungal, sarcoid, Kawasaki disease, et al
>    Neoplastic: Leukemia, lymphoma, neuroblastoma
>    Vascular: Vasculitis (collagen-vascular disease), HSP
>    Sore throat:
>    Infectious/inflammatory
>    Pharyngotonsillitis, bacterial, viral (all kinds), Stevens-Johnson, Kawasaki
>    Malignancy: leukemia/lymphoma


## Vomiting

Infectious, inflammatory (gastroenteritis)
>    Gastrointestinal obstruction
>    Neoplastic


## Rash

Infection/inflammatory (bacterial, viral, fungal), vasculitis, Kawasaki

Now, by the frequency of appearance in our groups, we may begin to prioritize. Unfortunately, at this time, it appears that GI obstruction can be eliminated, but all the others are still possible.

We now may invoke the epidemiologic aspect and prioritize by commonness of the conditions. Thus we may put the differential diagnosis categories in the following order:

Infectious/inflammatory

Vasculitis

Neoplastic

## TESTING THE HYPOTHESIS

At this point we have hypothesized several illnesses. When one tests a hypothesis, we are seeking further information to help determine whether or not this hypothesis is true. So the next step is to do a physical examination to gather more information that may eliminate some of the possibilities.

The only positive findings physical examination tells us that Ruthie has erythematous tonsils; a rash characterized by facial flush with circumoral pallor, a "strawberry-ish" tongue and has an odor about her mouth.

Thus, putting together a list at this point, we can lower the priority of inflammatory or malignancy for now because of the short duration of the illness, although we are not 100% sure. However, keep in mind that because the patient is stable, we have time to defer it for now.

## FURTHER TESTING OF THE HYPOTHESIS

At this point, we have generated a differential diagnosis, but do not have a certain answer. Minus the senior attending with his wealth of experience, the resident still may not be 100% certain of the diagnosis and, although he thinks it may be strep, he may need to test this hypothesis by performing a rapid strep antigen test. This is quite reasonable, as the test is neither costly nor potentially harmful.

## HEURISTICS

Heuristics is defined as: (taken from Wikipedia)

**Heuristic** (/hjʉˈrɪstɪk/; Greek: "Εὑρίσκω", **"find"** or **"discover"**) refers to experience-based techniques for problem solving, learning, and discovery that give a solution which is not guaranteed to be optimal. Where the exhaustive search is impractical, heuristic methods are used to speed up the process of finding a satisfactory solution via mental shortcuts to ease the cognitive load of making a decision. Examples of this method include using a rule of thumb, an educated guess, an intuitive judgment, stereotyping, or common sense.

In more precise terms, heuristics are strategies using readily accessible, though loosely applicable, information to control problem solving in human beings and machines.

Thus, heuristics are simply "short-cuts." Though imperfect, one must weigh their practicality against a tedious two-hour patient encounter. In a sense, even the "winnowing down" discussed above is a form of heuristics. It is true that "common things occur commonly." However, it is not totally impossible that on a given day, our patient may, unfortunately have a rare, more serious condition. Another good example of heuristics is pattern-recognition. Thus, in our case, the attending physician, with more experience has seen this constellation of findings many times and was able to recognize the diagnosis immediately.

A good example of a heuristic short-cut is the following story:

Two doctors were standing on a street corner. Coming into vision was a woman on the opposite side of the street. One of the doctors says. "I wonder what her diagnosis is. She seems to be about 75-80 years old, walks with a mild limp with her left arm held slightly flexed. I noticed she speaks with a middle European accent." The other doctor says: "Oh, that's my mother. She had a small bleed from an AVM two years ago." Thus, our experience definitely colors our knowledge and thought processes, and can be helpful in arriving at a correct answer.

The extreme form of pattern recognition is augenblick, German for "blink of the eye." You see it, you know it.


## PITFALLS IN DIAGNOSIS-DOWNSIDE OF HEURISTICS

We all must be mindful of heuristics that may lead us down an incorrect path. Some examples of pitfalls are:

## a. Availability

The tendency to make a judgment based on either the immediate availability of the given facts, or the availability of the facts in the clinician's mind based on his/her experience. Since we experience common things, they are more likely to come up first to the exclusion of other possibilities. Sometimes the availability error can go the other way. For example, if a doctor has been sued for having missed a certain diagnosis, this diagnosis may always be in the forefront of his/her mind and be invoked unnecessarily.

## b. Anchoring

Clinician does not consider other possibilities but firmly puts down anchor and unfortunately, in some cases may keep it there too long. It is always important to keep in mind at all times "What else can this be?"

## c. Logic vs. empiric data

Since we physicians fancy ourselves as "smarter than average," and have often used deductive logic to our benefit. In the real world one must look at the facts at hand (empirical data). Medicine, although an art, is still also an applied science.

## d. Escalation of commitment

The tendency to make decisions based on ones commitment put into the diagnosis. This type of fallacy is rampant in gamblers who think that the more they put into the pot, the more likely they may win (when to hold, when to fold). Another example is throwing good money after bad, or bidding wars at auctions. ("I have sunk so much into this, I must continue on.")

## e. Commission bias

Many doctors, especially surgeons and intensivists are driven by and have often succeeded with intervention. There is always a tendency to have to "do something," even if that will not always help.


## f. Attribution

Often a negative aspect of a patient's personality, even though true, will color the judgment of a physician performing an evaluation. As an example: the proverbial "crock." How many times have we rolled our eyes when we see a certain name on the patient roster? Have we already made up our mind that the patient is not sick this time?

Also the converse may be true. If we tend to be enamored of a patient, sometimes we will make an "affective error." We may like a patient so much and may act on our hope that he "really doesn't have cancer" and not perform a thorough enough investigation. This is a pitfall for the doctor who treats family members.


## g. Representativeness

Similar to attribution, a prototype of a patient may bias us. "How could a wiry 35 year old vegetarian non-smoker that runs marathons possibly be having a coronary?" However, to answer a question with another question: "Does every wiry 35 year-old vegetarian non-smoker that runs marathons always have to have the whole million-dollar cardiac workup?"


## h. Search satisfaction

Like the old joke: Q: "Where did you find your wallet." A: "In the last place I looked." This kind of satisfaction can lead to anchoring (see above).

## i. Yin-yang out

Tendency to think of many possibilities, not be able to come to a certain conclusion, then giving up. Not a good way to deal with uncertainty. Note the opposite; jumping to conclusions without testing the hypothesis, time permitting, is also problematic.


# SUMMARY

Clinical medicine can be a mine field. We constantly have to weigh practicality against time, cost, and potential untoward side effects.


## A slightly different twist to the case – a senior resident presentation

In this scenario, a second-year resident has seen the patient and has done the distillation process as presented above. **(Time elapsed: 7 min.)**


***Attending***
"So, what do you think is going on?"


***Resident***
Well, there are a few possibilities here. With the sore throat, fever and rash, the most common thing would be strep, but viral infections may also produce a similar picture. With the involvement of the oral mucosa one must also think of collagen vascular disorders, Stevens-Johnson syndrome and Kawasaki disease. I would put malignancy on a way-back burner and certainly would not mention it to the mom for fear of scaring the bejeebers out of her.


***Attending***
That's a reasonable differential. Don't think your tactfulness went by unnoticed. "She has a fever, her throat and tongue is kind of messy. It sounds more to me like a strep, enough to treat it now, but let's do a throat culture to be sure. We'll start her on penicillin 250 mg tid. Tell them to let us know if she isn't better in about a day or two." (Note this is a 2nd year resident so this case was "GE'd").

(Next day about 30 hours later, Ruthie's mom calls concerned that she still has a fever and that the rash is worsening. The schedule is full, but Dr. Senior tells the staff to work them in.)

***Attending***
"I'm a little worried that she isn't better. Typically strep responds in 24 hours. Also, the rash is now all over her palms and soles and her conjunctivae look slightly red with no exudates. I checked on the throat culture and it was negative."

(Attending and resident go into the room)

Ooh, this is a lot different from yesterday! I guess this turned out to be something else after all. Your differential diagnosis did include Kawasaki disease and now it has become more apparent. (To Ruthie and her mom): "I'm sorry, but this turned out to be something a little out of the ordinary. We are suspecting something else, and this needs to be evaluated and treated in the hospital. This may seem to be a bit more than you were expecting. Dr. Senior goes into explanation of Kawasaki disease at a level that Ruthie can understand.

(The clinic arranges for Ruthie's admission to the hospital for Kawasaki disease. The attending is self-flagellating with barbed wire as the curtain falls to the tune of the Beatles' "I'm a Loser.")

## Dénouement and discussion

Ruthie was admitted. Cardiology consult was obtained who felt it was either an early or an atypical Kawasaki. She had a normal echocardiogram with no evidence of coronary involvement. She responded nicely to a dose of IVIG and was discharged the next day. She defervesced and she is presently doing well.

Here is an example where an incorrect diagnosis was made. Note that the attending physician didn't go into the room this time. Did the resident not describe the rash perfectly? Was the attending physician too trusting? Did the rash really change?

However, the redeeming factor was that the error was picked up and corrected in a timely fashion. Scary, isn't it? Note that even though we are always treading in a mine field when we practice medicine, more so, academic medicine, we still are able, in most situations short of a calamity to think stepwise and reassess at all times.

N. B., always leave an opening for the patient to return if things do not go according to plan, even in a seemingly simple case!

# Chapter 4

# OVERDIAGNOSIS

Overdiagnosis is defined as making a diagnosis which is correct, but the knowledge of which may have little or no practicality. Acting on this knowledge could be to the detriment of the patient. Much of this has arisen as the result of multiple screening programs. There are many examples. Sometimes more questions than answers arise.

Screening adult men for prostate cancer – About 70% of men over age 75 have cancer cells in their prostates. It is a very slow-growing cancer. Should all men be screened and treated? Is screening of 40 year olds more appropriate than screening of 70 year olds?

Screening for coronary artery disease in an asymptomatic individual – Should a CABG be performed? Some "heart attacks" may present as sudden death. Will a CABG prevent this event? What if there is a therapeutic misadventure? Should research be directed toward identifying those who are more at risk for arrhythmia?

Similarly for universal screening mammograms for breast cancer – Studies have shown no real decrease in overall mortality. Should research be directed toward identifying those tumors with higher malignant potential?

Attention Deficit Disorder in children: Assuming the diagnosis is correct would more children benefit from properly administered behavior management and counseling?

Asymptomatic malrotation in a 14 year old – If a person has had this so many years, it is possible he/she will live a long life and die of something else? If this person is keenly aware of having this, and becomes symptomatic, most likely, timely diagnosis and surgery would work just fine. What if a person is on a cruise ship in the middle of the Pacific Ocean or visiting a third-world country and becomes symptomatic?

# Chapter 5

# WISDOM OBTAINED OVER THE YEARS

Summary of clinical aphorisms learned from my preceptors and life including hard knocks; navigating mines in the field.

- Facts vs. faith: Medicine is an art based on science (Osler)
- Treat the patient with the disease, not the other way around (Hippocrates, Osler)
- What do you want to know and when do you want to know it? (Howard Baker, Watergate scandal)
- Just because somebody, even a physician, tells you something, or you read a report, doesn't necessarily make it true (affective error)
- Lab tests test hypotheses, not patients
- Treat patients, not numbers. The best way to cure an abnormal lab test result in a normal patient is to repeat the test (commission bias)
- The best way to prevent an abnormal lab test result in a normal patient is not to have ordered it in the first place (commission bias)
- Barring a dire situation, just don't do something, stand there (commission bias)
- Common things occur commonly (availability)
- Things are seldom what they seem (Gilbert & Sullivan, HMS Pinafore, 1878 availability, representativeness)
- Never say "always"; never say 'never." Furthermore, don't even think them (anchoring)
- Always keep your mind open (yin-yang-out)
- Crazy people get sick, too (attribution). N. B. also, sick people can get crazy

- Know when to hold; know when to fold (commission bias)
- If the diagnosis or treatment plan is not going smoothly, reassess. Always be humble. Even the smartest clinicians make mistakes. The good ones recognize and recover from them (all of the above)
- If you cannot tolerate uncertainty, you certainly should not be practicing the art of medicine
- If you don't know what's going on, find someone who may
- If it ain't broke, don't always fix it now. If we can detect an abnormality in an asymptomatic individual, should we act on it now, later or never?
- A physician can be an imposing intimidating figure to a small child. Always keep in mind when doing a genital examination on a frightened two-year old: "How would I feel if somebody 15 feet tall were doing this to me?"

# Chapter 6

# ABOUT THE AUTHOR

Arthur N Feinberg, MD, FAAP is professor of Pediatrics and Adolescent Medicine at the Western Michgan University in Kalamazoo, Michigan, United States. He is also Professor of Pediatrics at the Michigan State University College of Human Medicine, Department of Pediatrics and Human Development, East Lansing, Michigan, as well as Clinical Professor of Pediatrics at the Michigan State University College of Osteopathic Medicine. He attended the Albert Einstein College of Medicine at the Yeshiva University in New York and completed pediatric internship and residency at Montefiore Hospital and Medical Center in New York. After serving two years in the US Navy he entered private practice in Kalamazoo in 1975. His strong interest in teaching led him to join the residency program in Kalamazoo in 1993. He has been recipient of six teaching awards since joining the faculty. His research interests have included newborn topics such as hospital discharge and circumcision and have led to several original publications and numerous book chapters. He has been co-editor of three textbooks. E-mail: arthur.feinberg@med.wmich.edu

# ABOUT THE DEPARTMENT OF PEDIATRIC AND ADOLESCENT MEDICINE, WESTERN MICHIGAN UNIVERSITY HOMER STRYKER MD SCHOOL OF MEDICINE (WMED), KALAMAZOO, MICHIGAN, UNITED STATES

## MISSION AND SERVICE

The Western Michigan University Homer Stryker M.D. School of Medicine was started in 2012 and its first class of medical students began in 2014. The Department of Pediatric and Adolescent Medicine has a pediatric residency program which is accredited by the Accreditation Council for Graduate Medical Education (ACGME) in Chicago, Illinois, USA and the current residency program in Pediatrics started in 1990.

The WMED Department of Pediatric & Adolescent Medicine has a commitment to a comprehensive approach to the health and development of the child, adolescent, and the family. The Department has a blend of academic general pediatricians and pediatric specialists. Our Pediatric Clinic team provides a broad spectrum of general well and sick child care (birth through 18 years) including immunizations, monitoring general physical and emotional growth, motor skill development, sports medicine (including participation evaluations and evaluation of common sports injuries), child abuse evaluations, and psychosocial or behavioral assessment. WMed Pediatrics believes in immunizations as a protection against preventative disease processes. Our Pediatrics Clinic is undergoing a transformation to a patient-centered medical home (PCMH). A patient-centered medical home is a way to deliver coordinated and comprehensive primary care to our infants, children, adolescents and young adults. It is a partnership between individuals and families within a health care setting, which allows for a more efficient use of resources and time to improve the quality of outcomes for all involved through care provided by a continuity care team.

## RESEARCH ACTIVITIES

The Department has a variety of research projects in adolescent medicine, neurobehavioral pediatrics, adolescent gynecology, pediatric diabetes mellitus, asthma, and cystic fibrosis. The WMED Department of Pediatric & Adolescent Medicine has published a number of medical textbooks: Essential adolescent medicine (McGraw-Hill Medical Publishers), The pediatric diagnostic examination (McGraw-Hill), Pediatric and adolescent psychopharmacology (Cambridge University Press), Behavioral pediatrics, 2nd Edition (iUniverse Publishers in New York and Lincoln, Nebraska), Behavioral Pediatrics 3rd Edition (New York: Nova Biomedical Books); 4th Edition: In Press. Pediatric practice: Sports medicine (McGraw-Hill), Handbook of Clinical Pediatrics (Singapore: World Scientific), Neurodevelopmental Disabilities: Clinical Care for Children and Young Adults (Dordrecht: Springer), Adolescent Medicine: Pharmacotherapeutics in Medical Disorders (Berlin/Boston: De Gruyter), Adolescent Medicine: Pharmacotherapeutics in General, Mental, and Sexual Health (Berlin/Boston: De Gruyter), Pediatric Psychodermatology (Berlin/Boston: De Gruyter), Substance Abuse in Adolescents and Young Adults: A Manual for Pediatric and Primary Care Clinicians (Berlin/Boston: De Gruyter), and Tropical Pediatrics (NY:Nova); Second Edition in Press.

The Department has edited a number of journal issues published by Elsevier Publishers covering pulmonology (State of the Art Reviews: Adolescent Medicine—AM:STARS), genetic disorders in adolescents (AM:STARS), neurologic/neurodevelopmental disorders (AM:STARS), behavioral pediatrics (Pediatric Clinics of North America), pediatric psychopharmacology in the 21st century (Pediatric Clinic of North America), nephrologic disorders in adolescents (AM:STARS), college health (Pediatric Clinics of North America), adolescent medicine (Primary Care: Clinics in Office Practice), behavioral pediatrics in children and adolescents (Primary Care: Clinics in Office Practice), adolescents and sports (Pediatric Clinics of

North America), and developmental disabilities (Pediatric Clinics of North America). The Department has also edited a journal issue on musculoskeletal disorders in children and adolescents for the American Academy of Pediatrics' AM:STARs; in April of 2013 a Subspecialty Update issue was published in AM:STARs.

The department has developed academic ties with a variety of international medical centers and organizations, including the Queen Elizabeth Hospital in Hong Kong, Indian Academy of Pediatrics (New Delhi, India), the University of Athens Children's Hospital (First and Second Departments of Paediatrics) in Athens, Greece and the National Institute of Child Health and Human Development in Jerusalem, Israel.

## Contact

Professor Donald E Greydanus, MD
Department of Pediatric and Adolescent Medicine
Western Michigan University Homer Stryker M.D. School of Medicine
1000 Oakland Drive, D48G, Kalamazoo, MI 49008-1284, United States
E-mail: Donald.greydanus@med.wmich.edu
and dilip.Patel@med.wmich.edu
Website: http://www.med.wmich.edu

# Chapter 8

# ABOUT THE BOOK SERIES "PEDIATRICS, CHILD AND ADOLESCENT HEALTH"

Pediatrics, child and adolescent health is a book series with publications from a multidisciplinary group of researchers, practitioners and clinicians for an international professional forum interested in the broad spectrum of pediatric medicine, child health, adolescent health and human development.

- Merrick J, ed. Child and adolescent health yearbook 2011. New York: Nova Science, 2012.
- Merrick J, ed. Child and adolescent health yearbook 2012. New York: Nova Science, 2012.
- Roach RR, Greydanus DE, Patel DR, Homnick DN, Merrick J, eds. Tropical pediatrics: A public health concern of international proportions. New York: Nova Science, 2012.
- Merrick J, ed. Child health and human development yearbook 2011. New York: Nova Science, 2012.
- Merrick J, ed. Child health and human development yearbook 2012. New York: Nova Science, 2012.
- Shek DTL, Sun RCF, Merrick J, eds. Developmental issues in Chinese adolescents. New York: Nova Science, 2012.
- Shek DTL, Sun RCF, Merrick J, eds. Positive youth development: Theory, research and application. New York: Nova Science, 2012.
- Zachor DA, Merrick J, eds. Understanding autism spectrum disorder: Current research aspects. New York: Nova Science, 2012.

- Ma HK, Shek DTL, Merrick J, eds. Positive youth development: A new school curriculum to tackle adolescent developmental issues. New York: Nova Science, 2012.
- Wood D, Reiss JG, Ferris ME, Edwards LR, Merrick J, eds. Transition from pediatric to adult medical care. New York: Nova Science, 2012.
- Isenberg Y. Guidelines for the healthy integration of the ill child in the educational system: Experience from Israel. New York: Nova Science, 2013.
- Shek DTL, Sun RCF, Merrick J, eds. Chinese adolescent development: Economic disadvantages, parents and intrapersonal development. New York: Nova Science, 2013.
- Shek DTL, Sun RCF, Merrick J, eds. University and college students: Health and development issues for the leaders of tomorrow. New York: Nova Science, 2013.
- Shek DTL, Sun RCF, Merrick J, eds. Adolescence and behavior issues in a Chinese context. New York: Nova Science, 2013.
- Sun J, Buys N, Merrick J, eds. Advances in preterm infant research. New York: Nova Science, 2013.
- Tsitsika A, Janikian M, Greydanus DE, Omar HA, Merrick J, eds. Internet addiction: A public health concern in adolescence. New York: Nova Science, 2013.
- Shek DTL, Lee TY, Merrick J, eds. Promotion of holistic development of young people in Hong Kong. New York: Nova Science, 2013.
- Shek DTL, Ma C, Lu Y, Merrick J, eds. Human developmental research: Experience from research in Hong Kong. New York: Nova Science, 2013.
- Merrick J, ed. Chronic disease and disability in childhood. New York: Nova Science, 2013.
- Rubin IL, Merrick J, eds. Break the cycle of environmental health disparities: Maternal and child health aspects. New York: Nova Science, 2013.
- Rubin IL, Merrick J, eds. Environmental health disparities in children: Asthma, obesity and food. New York: Nova Science, 2013.
- Rubin IL, Merrick J, eds. Environmental health: Home, school and community. New York: Nova Science, 2013.

- Rubin IL, Merrick J, eds. Child health and human development: Social, economic and environmental factors. New York: Nova Science, 2013.
- Merrick J, Kandel I, Omar HA, eds. Children, violence and bullying: International perspectives. New York: Nova Science, 2013.
- Omar HA, Bowling CH, Merrick J, eds. Playing with fire: Children, adolescents and firesetting. New York: Nova Science, 2013.
- Merrick J, Tenenbaum A, Omar HA, eds. School, adolescence and health issues. New York: Nova Science, 2013.
- Merrick J, Tenenbaum A, Omar Ha, eds. Adolescence and sexuality: International perspectives. New York: Nova Science, 2014.
- Diamond G, Arbel E. Adoption: The search for a new parenthood. New York: Nova Science, 2014.
- Taylor MF, Pooley JA, Merrick J, eds. Adolescence: Places and spaces. New York: Nova Science, 2014.
- Greydanus DE, Feinberg AN, Merrick J, eds. Born into this world: Health issues. New York: Nova Science, 2014.
- Greydanus DE, Feinberg AN, Merrick J, eds. Caring for the newborn: A comprehensive guide for the clinician. New York: Nova Science, 2014.
- Rubin IL, Merrick J, eds. Environment and hope: Improving health, reducing AIDS and promoting food security in the world. New York: Nova Science, 2014.
- Greydanus DE, Feinberg AN, Merrick J, eds. Pediatric and adolescent dermatology: Some current issues. New York: Nova Science, 2014.
- Roach RR, Greydanus DE, Patel DR, Merrick J, eds. Tropical pediatrics: A public helath concern of international proportions, Second edition. New York: Nova Science, 2015.
- Merrick J, ed. Child and adolescent health issues: A tribute to the pediatrician Donald E Greydanus. New York: Nova Science, 2015.

## Contact

Professor Joav Merrick, MD, MMedSci, DMSc
Medical Director, Medical Services
Division for Intellectual and Developmental Disabilities
Ministry of Social Affairs and Social Services
POBox 1260, IL-91012 Jerusalem, Israel
E-mail: jmerrick@zahav.net.il

# INDEX

## C

cancer, 3, 64, 69
cancer cells, 69
cervix, 33
chemosis, 18
Chicago, 75
child abuse, 75
childhood, 80
children, xi, 1, 2, 8, 21, 25, 69, 76, 80
circumcision, 73
classification, 58
clavicle, 35
clinical diagnosis, xiv
clinical experience, xi
clonus, 46
closure, 44
clubbing, 23, 24, 34
coffee, 45
cognitive function, 44
cognitive level, 1
cognitive load, 62
collagen, 60, 65
college students, 80
color, 19, 20, 21, 30, 31, 32, 49, 64
common sense, 59, 62
conduction, 45
confidentiality, 1, 7, 8
congenital heart disease, 24
connective tissue, 50
constipation, 2, 54
coronary artery disease, 69
cough, 24, 30
coughing, 54
counseling, 69
covering, 76
cracks, 50
cranial nerve, 45
culture, 65, 66
curriculum, 80
cyanosis, 24
cyanotic, 13, 23
cystic fibrosis, 76

## D

data collection, 53, 54
defects, 16
dementia, 5
deposits, 50
depression, 8
depth, 13, 22
dermatology, 81
dermis, 49, 50
destruction, 50, 59
detectable, 46
detection, 13, 20
deviation, 23
diabetes, 3, 76
diagnosis, xiii, xiv, 53, 56, 59, 60, 61, 62, 63, 66, 69, 72
diarrhea, 2, 54
diastolic pressure, 14, 15
diet, 3
differential diagnosis, 60, 61, 66
dilation, 18
direct observation, 18
disability, 5, 80
discharges, 31
discomfort, 13, 37, 43
discrimination, 47
dislocation, 35
disorder, 3, 59, 79
dissatisfaction, 4
distillation, xi, 65
distress, 12, 13, 22
distribution, 12
doctors, 62, 64
drainage, 20
drug consumption, 3
dyspnea, 54

## E

echocardiogram, 66
edema, 18, 24, 49
effusion, 35, 36
enamel, 21

endocrine, 3
environmental factors, 81
epidemiologic, 61
epidemiology, 59
epidermis, 50
equality, 18
erosion, 50
etiology, 58
evidence, 12, 66
evolution, xi
examinations, xiv
exercise, 3
exposure, 51, 55
extravasation, 50

## F

facial expression, 45
facies, 43
faith, 71
families, 76
family history, 55
family members, 3, 6, 64
fat, 12, 50
fear(s), 1, 6, 7, 65
feelings, 4, 5, 8
femur, 41
fever, 54, 56, 58, 59, 60, 65, 66
fibula, 41
flank, 28
flexibility, 35
fluctuant, 12, 16
fluid, 24, 25, 29, 31, 44, 50
food, 54, 55, 80, 81
food intake, 54
food security, 81
formation, 19, 21, 50
fremitus, 23
frenulum, 21

## G

gait, 34, 44, 48
gastroenteritis, 60

gastroenterologist, 55
genetic disorders, 76
geography, 6
Gestalt, 9, 12, 31, 32, 43
gestation, 55
gonorrhea, 56
gravity, 44, 48
Greece, 77
growth, 9, 15, 24, 44, 54, 75
gymnastics, 55
gynecomastia, 22

## H

hair, 35
headache, 54, 60
health, vii, ix, 2, 3, 8, 75, 76, 79, 80, 81
health care, 76
health status, 2
hearing impairment, 6
hearing loss, 45
heart attack, 69
heart rate, 25
height, 9, 12, 13
hematoma, 50
HIV, 55
HIV test, 55
homework, 8
Hong Kong, 77, 80
househusband, 55
human development, 79, 81
hypertension, 3
hypertrophy, 34, 35, 48

## I

iliac crest, 34, 36
immunization, 55
India, 77
induration, 16, 22, 35
infants, 21, 59, 76
infection, 50
inflammation, 50
ingestion, 54

## T





## U



## V

<table>
<tr><td>W</td><td>Y</td></tr>
</table>